Basic Medical Techniques
and
Patient Care
for
Radiologic Technologists

Basic Medical Techniques
and
Patient Care
for
Radiologic
Technologists

Lillian S. Torres, B.S., M.Ed.
Assistant Professor
Department of Allied Health
Chaffey College
Rancho Cucamonga, California

Carol Morrill Moore, A.R.R.T., B.V.E.
Assistant Professor
Department of Allied Health
Chaffey College
Rancho Cucamonga, California

J. B. Lippincott Company
PHILADELPHIA • TORONTO

ISBN 0-397-54222-4

Library of Congress Catalog Card Number 78-10520

Printed in the United States of America

4 6 8 9 7 5 3

Library of Congress Cataloging in Publication Data

Torres, Lillian S.
Basic medical techniques and patient care for
radiologic technologists.

Includes index.
1. Radiology, Medical. 2. Nursing.
3. Radiologic technologists. I. Moore, Carol
Morrill, joint author. II. Title.
RC78.T67   616.07'57   78-10520
ISBN 0-397-54222-4

Contents

Acknowledgments

We are most grateful to the radiologic technology students at Chaffey College who assisted and advised us while this text was being prepared. Their interest and cheerful cooperation will always be remembered.

Thanks also to:

Our colleagues at Chaffey College; particularly Mary Boul, Director of the Allied Health Department and Gordon Lockwood, RT who gave us their support and suggestions.

Janet A. Carey, RT, Administrator of Diagnostic Radiology, and Director, School of Radiologic Technology, Temple University Hospital, who reviewed the entire manuscript.

Aaron McDaniel, our photographer, who spent many hours working with us to obtain good photographic illustrations.

Rose Mary Spurling, our secretary.

Richard Steidl, M.D. and the radiology staff at Kaiser Foundation Hospital, Fontana, California.

The radiology staff and the nursing staff at San Antonio Community Hospital, Upland, California.

The radiology staff at Riverside General Hospital.

Finally, we wish to thank the J. B. Lippincott Company and particularly Bernice Heller, Editor, Health Sciences Division, for their interest and assistance given so graciously.

Lillian S. Torres
Carol Morrill Moore

Introduction

Radiologic technology has grown from a technical skill requiring a high school diploma and six months of apprenticeship in a radiology department into a skilled profession requiring at least three years of classwork and internship. Because it has become a profession and the RT has become a more prominent member of the health team, the expectations of the technologist's patients and associates are higher. The radiologic technologist is expected to have an increasing knowledge of the medical procedures performed in his department and an understanding of the patient as a human being who brings his emotional as well as his physical problems with him to the radiology department.

The RT is expected to recognize symptoms of emergency situations and know what action to take when they occur. He is expected to know how to control the spread of disease and how to create a surgically aseptic field when it is necessary in his department. He must also know how to conduct himself in the surgical suite, critical care division, emergency room, and hospital ward of any institution in which he is employed. The RT will be called upon to assist with medical procedures that require specific knowledge to be performed safely and without injury to him or to his patient.

Although the RT may not legally administer drugs, he will be called upon to assist with their administration. Any person who participates in any way in the administration of drugs must be properly instructed about the precautions, methods, and means of drug administration or he is a potential hazard in his department.

Teaching medical procedures to RT students is a relatively new idea and, although medical procedures and techniques are always basically the same, they require some adjustment when performed in the radiology area. This textbook is an adaptation of basic medical procedures and techniques to the radiology department.

Each chapter is written within a modular format, with a pre-post test in the Appendix at the end of the book. This particular format is used because of the varying degrees of medical knowledge that the RT student possesses. He may take the test before beginning each chapter and, if he demonstrates proficiency, proceed to the next chapter without delay.

Each chapter contains background material followed by specific directions for performance of medical procedures. It is the hope of the authors that the RT student will find this a useful preliminary text which will help him feel more confident in his own department and in other areas of the hospital.

The Radiologic Technologist and Patient Communication

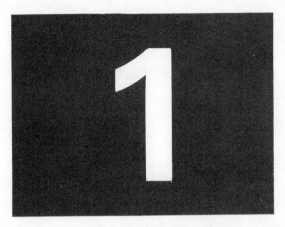

Goal of This Chapter

The RT must be aware that each patient who is sent to the radiology department brings his physical and emotional needs with him.

Objectives

When the student has completed this chapter, he will be able to:

1. List the basic physical needs of all patients.
2. List the basic psychological needs of all patients.
3. Describe threats to patient needs that may be present in the radiology department.
4. Assess the patient's general condition when he encounters him in the radiology department or on a hospital ward.
5. Describe problem-solving techniques in patient care.
6. List the RT's responsibility to his patients.
7. List the expectations a patient may have regarding the RT.
8. Explain the RT's ethical obligations to patients and colleagues.

Glossary

ambulatory able to walk about; not bedridden

anxiety painful or apprehensive uneasiness of mind often over anticipated illness

assess to make an evaluation of

Caucasian of or relating to the white race of mankind, classified according to physical features

emotional pertaining to feelings, appealing to or arousing emotion

deprivation a loss, often forcible or sudden

ethics a discipline dealing with good and bad and with moral duty

evaluation the act of determining the fixed worth of a product or human effort

All human beings have basic needs which govern their lives. Abraham Maslow, a renowned psychologist, felt that one was not able to advance to the proceeding stage in his social and psychological development if basic needs were not satisfied. Maslow's hierarchy of needs is as follows:

1. Physiologic needs: a person's basic needs are food, shelter, air, water, sleep, and sexual fulfillment. If these needs are not satisfied, one cannot pursue his other needs.
2. Safety and security: after the individual has satisfied his most basic needs, he begins to seek a place where he can be free from harm and sure of being able to earn a living for himself.
3. Love and belongingness: when primary needs are met, the person begins to seek someone with whom to share his life and a social group in which he feels accepted.
4. Self-esteem and the esteem of other human beings: every person thrives on his regard for himself and the feeling that he is favorably regarded by others beyond his immediate family or circle of significant others.
5. Self-actualization: when all of the foregoing needs have been met, the individual begins to grow spiritually. He begins to desire to accomplish deeds that will make him feel he has attained the ultimate growth in his life.

According to Maslow's hierarchy, one regresses when his needs are threatened. The sense of self-actualization is lost. Self-esteem and the esteem

Glossary cont.

health team   an organization with members from various professions, working cooperatively together in planning and giving total health care services

hierarchy   a ruling body organized in ranks or orders, each subordinate to the one above

nasogastric tube   a rubber or plastic tube inserted through the nose and down to the stomach

orthopedic   pertaining to the correction of deformities of bones or restoration of the function of the skeletal system

patient   a person who is ill or undergoing treatment for a disease

physiologic   conforming to the normal functioning of the body, a tissue or organ

profession   a calling requiring specialized knowledge and intensive academic preparation

psychological   having to do with mental processes

psychotic reaction   a behavior pattern of organic or emotional origin that elicits derangement of personality and loss of contact with reality

relate   to have or establish a relationship; interact with another person

self-actualization   realization of one's potential of intellectual growth

self-esteem   a high regard for one's self

standards   a model or example established by authority, custom, or general consent

timidity   absence of courage or self-confidence

unethical   against accepted standards of professional conduct

---

of others are gone. No longer is one loved or a part of a group. The sense of safety and security vanishes. These losses are so keenly felt that the individual again finds himself attempting to satisfy basic physiologic needs.

This is often the situation of a patient entering the radiology department. If he is seriously ill or fears that he might be, the threat is that much greater.

A patient who is to have a barium enema or a gastrointestinal series comes to the radiology department after having been deprived of food for at least twelve hours. He may have lost a night's sleep because of the series of enemas and cathartics he has had in preparation for his examinations. He has left the security of his home to endure this insult to his body. One cannot feel safe in the threatening environment of a radiology department, with its hard examining tables, windowless rooms, and mysterious equipment.

If the examination to be performed requires the insertion of a gastric tube or an injection, this can further lessen the patient's sense of comfort and safety. When a person does not feel physically secure, and the normal need for food, water, and sleep has not been satisfied, he begins to feel threatened emotionally.

When the medical diagnosis is uncertain, there is always cause for fear and questions. "Will I have a problem that requires surgery? Will the doctor discover that I have the malignant tumor I fear I have?"

Confirmation of serious illness or even mild anxiety about one's health can cause worry and uncertainty about the future. A young man with a family will be concerned about his family's financial support if he is ill. A young woman may fear losing her husband's love if she is found to have an illness that requires disfiguring surgery. Any person who is a patient is in some way threatened by what is about to happen. Consequently, the RT often sees the patient at one of the lowest points in that person's life—when the basic physiologic and psychological needs have been threatened.

A person in this condition may not behave logically or rationally. The patient has submitted himself for treatment by a hospital staff and cannot escape his menacing environment. He may react emotionally by becoming overly aggressive or by withdrawing emotionally from the unpleasant situation.

The RT must consider the patient's disturbed state when admitting him for examination or treatment. He must remember that the patient is not able to function at his best, and must do everything possible to reassure and comfort the patient while providing care. This is not an easy task; the RT often is faced with an aggressive or a withdrawn person to whom it is difficult to relate. The RT must be able to accept every patient as a unique individual who, in spite of temporary unpleasant behavior, is entitled to humane treatment provided in a dignified manner.

But before the RT can relate well to patients, he must understand himself and have his own needs satisfied. He should know his own strengths and weaknesses and not let them interfere with his work. He must be able to accept and respect himself. An RT who is physically ill or emotionally disturbed cannot cope satisfactorily with patients.

RT's Responsibility to Patients

One of the RT's primary responsibilities to patients is to look presentable and feel well every day. He should be well rested and free of disease. His uniform should be clean, and he must bathe daily. Personal problems should not interfere with patient care. Patient needs must be given first priority.

Every person who requires care expects a certain level of performance from the provider. When the RT greets the patient, the patient believes he is entrusting himself to the care of an educated and trained professional. He expects that person to demonstrate skill in doing his work. He also expects that person to perform his duties thoughtfully and treat the patient in an understanding and accepting way.

Every patient should be assured of as much physical privacy as is possible while the radiographic treatments are in progress. Each step of every procedure should be explained to the patient at the level of his understanding before it is begun. The RT will soon discover that if he is honest in his explanations and expectations, patients usually will be less fearful and more eager to cooperate. Treatment provided in a vague, impersonal fashion can give rise to fear and apprehension. This makes patient cooperation more difficult to obtain.

Evaluating the Patient's Needs

When the patient is received into the radiology department, the RT assigned to his care must be able to make a rapid mental assessment of the patient's condition and the special needs that person may have while in his care. This must be done systematically. If it is not made a preliminary to each radiographic procedure, the work will not proceed smoothly. Every problem will present itself as a separate entity, and the work in progress will have to be stopped while the problem is solved.

For the RT's purposes this patient assessment or evaluation may be divided into three sections: physical, emotional, and cultural.

THE PHYSICAL ASSESSMENT

After greeting the patient, the RT must observe him for a moment, seeking external clues that the patient will unconsciously provide. These clues can be very helpful to the technologist as he reflects upon the information he has gathered which will indicate the number and types of problems a particular patient may present.

First, observe the patient's grooming. If he is an outpatient, are his clothes clean and well pressed or are they dirty and unkempt? Does the patient look and smell clean? Is his hair combed? Are his teeth clean and do they appear to be cared for? A patient who has an unkempt appearance is often too physically or emotionally ill to perform the usual tasks of grooming.

Thus, an untidy appearance is your first clue that this patient may have a problem that could make caring for him more difficult.

Next, observe the patient's posture and ability to move. If he is an ambulatory patient, does he stand erect, or is he bent or slumped over? Does he walk easily, or does he appear to find ambulation difficult? Does he complain of pain in a particular part of his body? If he does not complain of pain, does he appear to be protecting a limb or an area of his body when he moves?

If the patient is in a wheelchair or on a gurney, you will have to rely on the information contained in his chart about his mobility. You might want to question the patient directly about it. Be certain before you ask a patient to move that he is able to do so without causing further injury or pain. If he is unable to move safely by himself, you will have to summon extra help.

It is also important to take notice of the patient's skin color and manner of breathing. Does he breathe quietly and without apparent difficulty, or are his respirations labored? If the patient is Caucasian, is his skin color pale, or does it have a bluish or gray tinge that might indicate respiratory or circulatory problems? If the patient is black or Chicano, it might be necessary to check fingernail beds or the mucous membrane of the mouth to ascertain whether there is a circulatory impairment. Bluish nail beds and mucous membranes are indicative of circulatory disturbance.

Are the patient's sensory capacities within normal limits? Does he respond normally to your questions without asking that a question be repeated or that you speak louder? Either of these responses might indicate hearing loss. Uncertainty of movement might indicate that the patient does not see clearly.

THE EMOTIONAL ASSESSMENT

Simply to enter a radiology department as an outpatient for a very simple radiographic examination may be anxiety-producing. To the patient who has, or fears that he may have, a serious illness, presenting himself for a diagnostic examination may produce severe anxiety. The RT is familiar with the surroundings of the radiology department and may not realize why the patient's behavior is as it is. He must learn to anticipate and recognize symptoms of anxiety so that he can help ease the patient's anxiety. Mild anxiety may be expressed as timidity, apprehension, or indecisiveness. As it becomes more severe, the patient may perspire or may have difficulty breathing. He may be either extremely restless or unable to move without being prodded. The anxious person's behavior may be very hostile or very aggressive; or he may be totally unresponsive.

Occasionally, severe trauma or illness may produce a psychotic reaction. This might display itself in bizarre behavior such as speaking to persons who are not present, laughing inappropriately, crying, and so on. Often a patient is concerned and anxious because a previous medical treatment caused him some difficulty. If a patient tells you that he has had problems during previous treatment, do not discount the information.

As the RT moves through the rapid assessment process, he must make accurate observations about his patient's behavior because it will affect his manner of treatment. If the patient is extremely anxious, the RT will need to spend more time preparing the patient for treatment than would be the case if the patient were relaxed and cooperative.

THE CULTURAL ASSESSMENT

The RT must be cognizant of the way in which a patient's cultural background affects his acceptance of treatment. Usually people who have been born and raised in the United States are reasonably accepting of prescribed treatment or examination in the radiology department. However, a person who has been raised in another culture might be extremely wary or hostile when he arrives in the radiology department for the first time. Cultural differences must be observed and noted in the process of assessment because they also may influence the patient's receptivity to treatment.

Problem Solving

When the RT is assigned to a particular patient, he must decide how he can perform the assigned task quickly, efficiently, and as comfortably for the patient as possible. List and consider the data that have been gathered: e.g., the patient is unable to stand on his left foot; the patient is hostile; or the patient is uncooperative. Irrelevant data are disregarded. The RT must consider his goal and the problems that may be encountered before that goal is achieved. Various plans of action must be considered. Evaluate each one, and decide which one will best suit the particular situation. If each assignment is dealt with in a systematic way, the RT will be able to accomplish the goal set for each patient in the minimum amount of time and with the best results for both patient and technologist.

Medical Ethics

As the RT student becomes more familiar with the routines of the hospital and particularly those of the radiology department, he will begin to work with more comfort and ease. He must always remember the ethics of his profession.

As a professional person, the RT has a duty to cooperate with his medical co-workers. He must try to accommodate not only patients, but all the nurses, doctors, and fellow RTs also involved in patient care. It is unethical for an RT to reveal to anyone not professionally involved in the care of a patient the patient's name or the procedures performed. This prohibition extends to relatives and friends of the patient. If there are questions about the nature of a patient's treatment or diagnosis to be answered, the questioner may be referred to the department radiologist.

It is also unethical for the RT to offer criticism of doctors, nurses, or other team members to any patient or any other person outside the hospital. If the RT is the observer of unethical or illegal practice in his department, it is his duty to report such practice to the proper person (usually the department head). If this is not effective, he should present the matter to his professional organization for discussion.

The RT must be continually aware of himself as a member of a professional health team and must work to improve the standards of his profession. He can do this by always maintaining the high standards of practice that he learns as a student and by seeking methods of raising these standards whenever the opportunity presents itself.

Summary

The RT must recognize that each patient who arrives in the radiology department for care has physical and emotional needs which are threatened by illness. It is his duty as a professional person to provide assurance and comfort to his patients by his manner of relating to them and by his work competence. He must learn to assess each patient and anticipate problems that may arise before he undertakes care. This ensures uninterrupted, competent treatment. He must also remember that he is a professional person and that professional standards of ethics must be maintained. The RT must respect the patient's right to confidentiality and must respect and cooperate with his co-workers.

See Appendix for pre-post test on Chapter 1.

Medical Asepsis in the Radiology Department

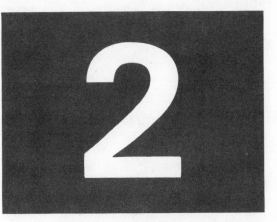

Goal of This Chapter

The RT must assume personal responsibility for controlling the spread of microorganisms in the radiology department.

Objectives

When the student has completed this chapter, he will be able to:

1. List four common means by which microorganisms are spread in the radiology department.
2. Define the terminology used in this chapter.
3. Give a laboratory demonstration of three methods of controlling the spread of microorganisms by means of good medical aseptic technique.

Glossary

aerobe   a microorganism that lives and grows in the presence of oxygen

anaerobe   a microorganism that cannot live in the presence of oxygen

antibiotic   a chemical substance produced by a microorganism which has the capacity, in dilute solution, to inhibit growth of or to kill other microorganisms

antiseptic   a substance used to destroy pathogenic organisms

asepsis   the prevention of contact with microorganisms

bacteriostatic   a substance that prevents the growth of microorganisms

communicable   capable of being transmitted from one person to another

contaminate   to make unclean; to introduce microorganisms into an area where they had not previously been present

direct contact   actual touching of a person with a communicable disease

Radiologic technologists are responsible for preventing the spread of microorganisms in their department. This can be accomplished by practicing good medical aseptic technique. Medical asepsis is any practice which helps reduce the number and spread of microorganisms; therefore, it involves the proper cleaning of any article that contains microorganisms or harbors them on its surface.

It was once thought that only certain specific microorganisms caused disease. Recently it has been discovered that almost any microorganism in any area other than its natural environment may be the cause of infection or disease. For example, *Escherichia coli*, which normally inhabits the human intestinal tract, will not cause disease in that location; however, should it gain entrance to the urinary bladder it can cause a urinary tract infection. For this reason it is necessary that the RT, as a member of the health team, consider all microorganisms as potentially pathogenic. He should endeavor constantly to reduce their numbers or eliminate them by practicing medical asepsis at all times.

There is a difference between medical asepsis and surgical asepsis. Medical asepsis means that, insofar as possible, microorganisms have been eliminated through use of soap, water, friction, and various other agents. Surgical asepsis means that microorganisms and their spores have been totally destroyed by means of heat or a chemical process.

In the daily routine of the radiology department, it is not practical or necessary to practice surgi-

Glossary cont.

disinfect to destroy pathogens, but not necessarily to destroy spores

disinfectant a substance used to destroy pathogens; in general, used on objects rather than on human beings

droplet infection a spray of mist containing pathogenic microorganisms ejected from the nose or mouth when coughing, sneezing, or talking

gram-negative losing the stain or being decolorized by alcohol in Gram's method of staining; a primary characteristic of certain microorganisms

gram-positive retaining the stain or resisting decoloration by alcohol in Gram's method of staining; a primary characteristic of some microorganisms

indirect contact touching objects contaminated by infected persons

infectious caused by or capable of being communicated by infection

medical asepsis practice that reduces the number and spread of microorganisms

microorganism a tiny living animal or plant visible only with a microscope

pathogen a disease-producing microorganism

spore a cell produced by a microorganism which under favorable conditions develops into an active microorganism

staphylococcus (plural staphylococci) microorganisms of the family Micrococcaceae that are the commonest cause of localized suppurative infections

sterilization the complete removal of microorganisms and spores

---

cal asepsis at all times, but one must always adhere to good medical asepsis. The RT does this to protect patients from contracting any communicable disease he may have as well as to protect himself from contracting a communicable disease from a patient.

Medical asepsis is part of our daily lives. In our homes we bathe, clean our eating utensils, eliminate dust, and so on. These are all methods of protecting ourselves from becoming ill due to the possible presence of disease-producing microorganisms. There are also governmental rules that protect us from certain diseases. Before an immigrant is allowed to enter the United States, he must show proof of inoculation against communicable diseases. There are federal pure food and drug laws that apply throughout the country; and public health departments in every community make every possible effort to control the spread of communicable diseases.

In hospitals, the fight to control disease is an ongoing one. Showers, tubs, and other patient bathing areas are cultured routinely. One newborn nursery is emptied, cleaned, and kept vacant for six weeks while another is used. Operating rooms are washed thoroughly with antiseptic solutions after each use. If a patient is suspected of having a communicable disease, he is immediately isolated. Every member of the medical team, from maintenance personnel to physicians, is constantly reminded of the need to practice good medical asepsis. The RT is no exception to this rule even though his particular situation may make it more difficult to remember.

Persons arrive in the radiology department from different environments, so the possibility that microorganisms will be spread is perhaps even greater here than elsewhere in the hospital. Though some arriving patients appear to be in good health, all patients must be regarded as potential carriers of disease. Every piece of equipment must be thoroughly cleaned after each use, and the RT must try to protect himself from infection.

How Microorganisms Are Spread

To contaminate means to render unclean. With reference to medical asepsis, an area or piece of equipment is considered contaminated if it is believed to harbor disease-producing microorganisms. A microorganism has basic requirements for survival, including warmth, food, and water or moisture. Some microorganisms need oxygen; these are called aerobes. Others, called anaerobes, cannot live in the presence of oxygen. Tetanus and gangrene are the best-known diseases caused by anaerobic microorganisms. Some microorganisms produce cells which are called spores. These are similar in some ways to eggs in that they have a kind of "coat" which protects them from heat, cold, and dryness and compensates for the lack of nourishment. This protective coat makes destruction of spores very difficult, and under favorable conditions they develop into active microorganisms. Thus, a patient or an RT with a broken area in the skin—especially a deep wound—is highly vulnerable to spores which become embedded in the wound and, when circumstances are favorable, begin to grow. Unbroken skin is usually resistant to spores.

Microorganisms thrive in damp, dark areas where there is little air circulation. Obviously, their growth is deterred in an area that is kept dry, light, and airy, especially if it is exposed to sunlight. Hence one of the best methods of controlling microorganisms is keeping the working areas dry and well lighted, and the ventilating system in good working order.

For present purposes, it may be stated that microorganisms are transmitted in four main ways. These will be discussed in a later chapter, but for the present the RT should keep in mind that contact with an area of infection or an infected person is the most common means of spread. The contact may be direct, by actually touching a person with a communicable disease or an area of infection; or it may be indirect, by touching objects that have been contaminated by disease (such as surgical instruments, dressings, and tissues). Contact may also occur by droplet infection, that is, infection of a person through spray or mist ejected from an infected person's nose or mouth when he coughs or sneezes.

These modes of transmission are often referred to as "the cycle of infectivity"; if the cycle is interrupted and broken, then infection can be controlled. The members of the health team must make every effort to break the cycle. For instance, if a patient with an obvious upper respiratory infection, such as a cold, is coughing or sneezing, be sure that he is provided with tissues and is instructed to cough and sneeze *into* these. Upper respiratory infections are spread by droplet infection; hence coughing into the tissues will stop the spread of the disease.

Other methods of stopping the spread of microorganisms that can be employed by the RT are: proper handwashing before and after handling supplies and after giving care to each patient; handling all patient body discharges as if they contain disease-producing microorganisms, and properly discarding them; proper cleaning of equipment used for patients and proper disposal of disposable items. Breaks or cracks in the RT's skin should be covered with sterile dressings. Spilling or splashing liquids on clothing should be avoided. The RT should wear no jewelry other than a wristwatch while on duty, as such articles harbor microorganisms. If there is any doubt about the cleanliness of an item, it should not be used.

In spite of all efforts to keep the environment medically aseptic, spread of disease to susceptible persons can occur. The RT will be doing himself, his co-workers, and his patients a great service if he keeps himself well rested and in good health. These measures will make him less susceptible to infectious disease.

Many persons wrongly believe there is no need to be concerned that they may spread disease-causing microorganisms. They reason that good medical asepsis is not always necessary because there is an antibiotic to cure every disease. This line of reasoning is false, and the medical worker who follows it and whose medical aseptic technique is deficient is guilty of providing poor care and is doing patients and co-workers an injustice.

There are many organisms against which antibiotics are ineffective. Among them are most viruses and the staphylococcus (often called staph), a gram-positive bacterium which does not cause any single identifiable disease but is responsible for numerous infections. Hospitals are particularly good breeding grounds for staph organisms, and once these organisms gain a foothold, they can do endless damage. The organism causes boils, styes, and food poisoning. Also, it is a frequent cause of surgical wound infections. Staph is spread by direct contact, and no antibiotic that is effective against it has yet been found.

Cleaning and Proper Disposal of Waste

The RT should follow these rules when disposing of wastes or cleaning equipment after patient use in the radiology department:

1. Flush away contents of bedpans or urinals promptly unless they are being saved for diagnostic specimen.
2. Rinse bedpans and urinals and send them to the proper place (usually a central supply area) for sterilization if they are not to be used for the same patient a second time.
3. Use equipment and supplies for one patient only. After the patient leaves the area, the supplies must be destroyed or re-sterilized before being used again.
4. Keep water and supplies clean and fresh. In the radiology department it is best to use paper cups and dispose of them after a single usage.
5. Floors are heavily contaminated. If an item that is to be used for a patient falls to the floor, discard it or send it to the proper department to be re-cleaned.
6. Avoid raising dust because it can carry microorganisms. When cleaning, use a cloth thoroughly moistened with a disinfectant.
7. When cleaning an article such as a radiographic table, start with the least soiled area and progress to the most soiled area. This prevents cleaner areas from becoming more heavily contaminated. Use a good disinfectant cleaning agent.
8. Place dampened or wet items such as dressings and bandages in waterproof bags and close the bags tightly before discarding them to prevent the handlers of this material from coming in contact with body discharges.
9. Do not re-use rags or mops for cleaning until they have been properly disinfected and dried.
10. Pour liquids to be discarded directly into a drain or toilet. Avoid splashing or spilling them.
11. If in doubt about the cleanliness or sterility of an item, *do not use it*.

Handwashing for Medical Asepsis

Of all the procedures one can follow to prevent the spread of microorganisms, none is more important than handwashing. In fact, many authorities believe that the hands are responsible for most spread of infection. This is why health team members are constantly being reminded of the necessity of handwashing.

The RT must be particularly careful to wash his hands after caring for each patient, as well as when handling equipment and dressings used in the course of individual patient care. There is a specific handwashing technique that is accepted as medically aseptic and that must be followed by the RT when working in the radiology department. This technique must not be confused with the surgical scrub, which will be described in another chapter. The medically aseptic handwashing technique is as follows:

1. Approach the sink. Do not allow your uniform to touch the sink because the sink is considered contaminated.

2. Turn on the tap; a sink with foot or knee controls is most desirable but is not always available. If the faucet is turned on by hand, use a paper towel to touch the handles and then discard the towel.

3. Regulate the water to a comfortably warm temperature.

4. Regulate the flow of water so that it does not splash from the sink.

5. During the entire procedure, keep your hands and forearms lower than your elbows. The water will drain by gravity from the areas of least to the areas of greatest contamination.

6. Wet the hands and soap them well. Liquid soap is most convenient, but often only bar soap is available. When using bar soap, rinse the bar before using it and hold it during the entire procedure. The soap dish is considered contaminated; if the soap bar is replaced during the procedure and then re-used, the hands will be re-contaminated.

7. With a firm circular rubbing motion, wash the palms of the hands, the backs of the hands, each finger, between the fingers, and finally the knuckles.

8. Rinse the hands well under running water.

9. Wet the wrists and forearms to the elbows. Apply soap and rub with the same circular motion, and then drop the soap into the soap dish. Do not touch the soap dish.

10. Rinse, allowing the water to run down over the hands.

11. Clean the fingernails with a brush or an orange stick carefully each day before beginning work and again if the hands become heavily contaminated.

12. Rinse the fingers well under running water.

13. If the hands become heavily contaminated during the work day, they should be scrubbed with a disposable brush.

14. Repeat washing procedure as described above.

15. Rinse the soap well and replace it in the dish. Do not touch the sink or the soap dish.

16. Turn off the water. If the handles are hand operated, use a paper towel to turn them off to avoid contamination of the hands.

17. Dry the arms and hands using as many towels as are necessary to do the job well.

18. Use lotion frequently on the hands and forearms. It helps keep the skin from cracking, and therefore helps prevent infection. (See Figs. 2-1, 2-2, 2-3, 2-4, and 2-5.)

The foregoing procedure should be performed at the beginning of each working day and any time the RT knows that his hands have been heavily contaminated. Wash hands in a similar manner between patients and at intervals, being careful not to touch the sink or faucet handles. Practicality will not allow time for such a long scrub every few minutes.

Summary

As part of the hospital medical team the RT has the responsibility of following strict medical aseptic technique. The term medical asepsis means the practice of keeping oneself, the equipment one handles, and the department in which one works as clean and free of microorganisms as possible without resorting to sterilization procedures.

Microorganisms can be spread by direct or indirect contact or by droplet contact. They are transmitted in a cycle of infectivity, and it is the RT's responsibility to break the cycle by practicing good medical aseptic technique.

The medical aseptic techniques to be employed in the radiology department include proper handwashing after caring for each patient and after handling contaminated supplies. Soiled dressings and discharges from patients must be properly discarded. Thorough cleaning of equipment after use by each patient, care in handling soiled linens, and proper disposal of disposable items are also necessary. However, proper handwashing is the most effective of all the techniques employed in medical asepsis in controlling the spread of microorganisms.

It must be remembered that depending on antibiotics to control disease is considered poor practice. These agents are not effective in the control of most viral and staphylococcal infections.

See Appendix for pre-post test on Chapter 2.

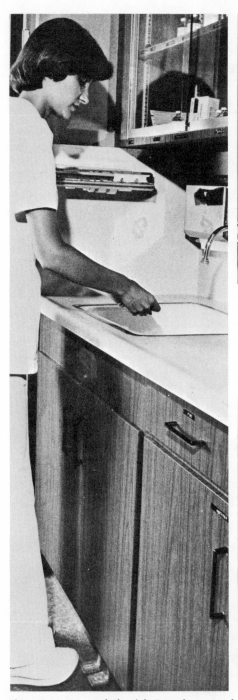

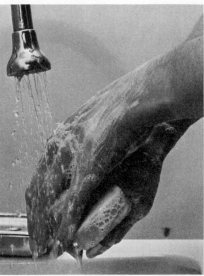

Figure 2-2. Your hands, knuckles, and areas between your fingers are cleaned with a firm rubbing motion. Continue to hold the soap while doing this. Figures 2-2 through 2-5 are from LuVerne Wolff Lewis, *Fundamental Skills in Patient Care* (Philadelphia: J.B. Lippincott Company, 1976), pp. 48–50.

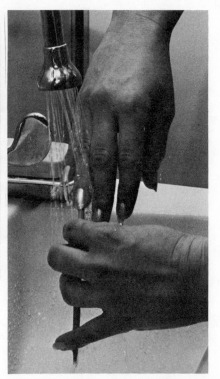

Figure 2-4. Clean your fingernails under running water to flush away dirt and microorganisms.

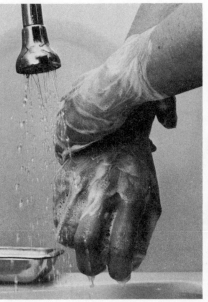

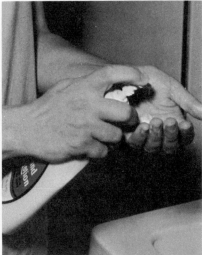

Figure 2-1. Approach the sink. Turn the tap, and adjust the water temperature. Stand away from the sink so that your uniform does not become contaminated. Wet hands and forearms.

Figure 2-3. Clean your wrists and forearms with a firm, circular motion. Then drop the soap into the soap dish.

Figure 2-5. Apply lotion to prevent chapping and cracking.

Admitting the Patient to the Radiology Department

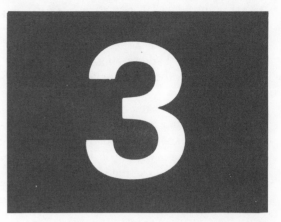

3

Goal of This Chapter

The RT student must be able to assist patients in dressing and undressing and must take responsibility for the care of their belongings while they are in the radiology department.

Objectives

When the student has completed this chapter he will be able to:

1. Give clear oral instructions to ambulatory patients about the correct manner of dressing or undressing for an x-ray examination.
2. Give a written explanation of what he should do to protect patients' belongings while they are in the radiology department.
3. Demonstrate in the laboratory situation the proper method of dressing or undressing a disabled patient for an x-ray examination.
4. Demonstrate in the laboratory situation the correct manner of assisting a patient with a bedpan or urinal, to make the patient comfortable and assure him privacy, with medically aseptic technique.

Glossary

bedpan a vessel for receiving the urinary or fecal discharges of a patient unable to leave his bed

brace an orthopedic appliance used to support a body part

contracture a state of permanent flexion of joints or muscles due to disease or degeneration of muscle or bony tissue

defecate to evacuate fecal material from the rectum

distal remote, farther from any point of reference

draw sheet a small sheet placed under the

When an outpatient comes to the radiology department, he is frequently required to remove all or some items of clothing before a radiologic examination can be performed. The RT will usually be the one who receives the patient and informs him which items of clothing are to be removed. The patient's discomfort or embarrassment can be lessened if the RT will approach the situation in a courteous and professional manner.

When the patient arrives for his examination, he should be taken to the specific place where he is expected to disrobe. The RT shows the patient how to close the dressing room door or draw the curtain of the cubicle while he is undressing. He should clearly explain how the patient is to don the examination gown and where he is to go for the examination after he is dressed in the examining gown. Doing this will take only a few moments of the RT's time and will make the patient feel more relaxed. Remember that everyone does not know that some types of examining gowns open at the back rather than at the front—it helps to be given an explanation.

Many patients bring jewelry, a purse, or other valuables to the radiology department. The dressing rooms in most radiology departments are not safe places to leave these items, and the patient will feel uneasy about leaving them there. Again, the RT should consider the patient's concerns and explain what he is to do with his clothing and valuables.

The patient should be supplied with hangers for his clothing. If it is permissible for him to leave his

Glossary cont.

trunk of the body for added protection or to facilitate moving a patient

extremity an arm or a leg, sometimes applied specifically to a hand or a foot

fasting going without food or drink for a given period of time

Fowler's position patient's upper body and head elevated 45° in a sitting position

fracture pan a specially shaped bedpan that is flattened and that has a wide lip in the back for patients who are unable to use the regular bedpan

intravenous (IV) within a vein

lavatory a room for washing; it contains one or more toilets

paralysis loss or impairment of motor function in a part due to injury or disease

perineum the pelvic floor and the structures occupying the pelvic outlet

peristalsis the wormlike movements by which the digestive tract propels its contents

supine lying on the back, face upward

urinal a vessel or other receptacle for urine

urinate to void or discharge urine

proximal nearest; closer to a point of reference

---

clothing in the dressing room, this fact should be explained by the RT. If it is not, the patient should be shown where he may leave his clothing. Purses, jewelry, and other valuables should be treated with special care.

Care of Valuables

Metal items such as necklaces, rings, and watches are not to be worn for certain radiographic examinations and must be removed before the examination is begun. An envelope large enough to accommodate all such items should be offered to the patient. The envelope may be kept in the patient's purse or pocket or in a secure place in the radiology department. This precaution also applies to billfolds and purses. If items are not to be carried by the patient, his name should be carefully written on a receipt along with other identifying information, and the items should be tagged and placed in a designated safety area by the RT. This procedure will prevent losses which may cause inconvenience and expense to both the patient and the department. The RT should never place a value on a patient's belongings—an item that may seem insignificant to the RT may be the patient's most treasured belonging. Each article of clothing, jewelry, or other personal effects that a patient brings to the radiology department should be treated as valuable.

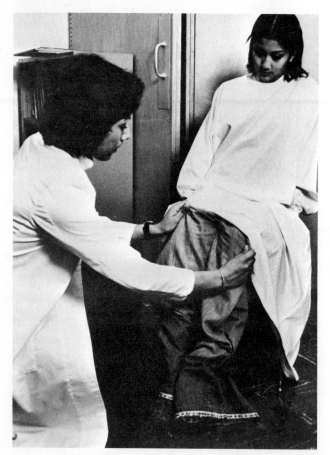

Figure 3-1

Assisting the Outpatient to Dress and Undress

The patient may arrive at the radiology department alone. As the RT is making his initial assessment of the patient's condition, he may observe that the person will need help in removing his clothing. This assistance would be necessary if the patient is in a cast or a brace or is too young or in too weakened a condition to help himself. He may have a contracture of an extremity. His eyesight may be poor. Whatever the problem, if the RT senses that the patient will have difficulty undressing if left alone, he should offer assistance and stay near the patient's dressing room to provide help when it is needed.

Occasionally a patient is brought to the radiology department as an emergency case. Removing his clothing in the conventional way may cause further injury or pain. The RT might consider cutting the garments away, but must not cut any item of clothing without gaining the patient's consent. If the patient is unable to give consent, a member of his family should do so in writing for the RT's protection.

If the patient is very young and is accompanied by a familiar adult, he will be more relaxed and cooperative if the adult helps him to dress and undress. Explain to the adult how the child should be dressed for the examination, arrange a meeting place and leave them alone.

If the RT must assist a patient who has a paralyzed leg or a leg or hip disability to undress, the clothing should be removed from the top part of the body first. Then place a long examining gown on the patient. Instruct him to loosen belt buckles, buttons, or hooks around the waist and slip the clothing over his hips. If the patient cannot do this for himself, the RT must reach under the gown and pull the clothing down over the hips. Then have the patient sit down. The RT can squat in front of the patient and gently pull the clothing over his legs and feet to remove it (Fig. 3-1).

Some dresses may be removed in this way. If it is not practical, and the dress must be pulled over the woman's head, the RT should place a draw sheet over her and then help her to remove her slip and bra. Help her to put on an examining gown, then remove the draw sheet.

To re-dress a patient with a paralyzed leg, or one with a leg injury or a leg cast or brace, slide the clothing over his feet or legs, as far as his hips, while he is wearing an examining gown and is in a sitting position. Then have the patient stand, and pull the clothing over his hips if he can tolerate this. If the patient is not able to pull his clothing over his hips by himself, the RT should have an assistant raise the patient off the chair so that the clothing may be slipped over the hips and to the waist. Then remove his arms from the sleeves of the gown; while he holds the gown over his chest, carefully pull the items over his head or put a shirt on him one sleeve at a time. When the outside items of clothing are on him, pull the gown out from under the clothes.

If a patient with an arm injury needs assitance to dress or undress, remove clothing from the unaffected side first. Next remove the clothing from the affected side, using the clean gown or a draw sheet to cover the chest. Then put the clean gown on the affected side first. Do not leave a patient unnecessarily exposed when assisting him to dress and undress (Fig. 3-2).

The Disabled Patient

If a patient is on a gurney or the radiographic table and the RT must change his clothing, this will be most easily accomplished with the patient in a supine

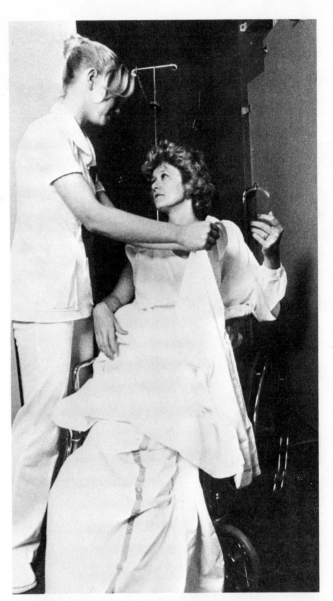

Figure 3-2.   Do not leave the patient exposed when assisting him (her) to dress or undress.

position. Cover him with a draw sheet and have an examining gown ready for use. Explain what is to be done and ask the patient to help if he is able. If he is paralyzed or unconscious, summon help before beginning the procedure.

Remove the clothing from the less affected side first. Next, remove the clothing from the affected side and place the clean gown on the affected side. Keep the patient covered with a draw sheet while doing this. Next place the clean gown on the unaffected side. Tie the gown at the back if this is practical (Fig. 3-3).

If the patient is wearing an item of clothing that must be pulled over his head, roll the garment up above the waist. Then remove the patient's arms from the clothing, first from the unaffected side and then

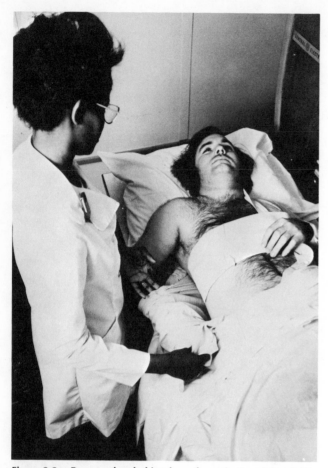

Figure 3-3.   Remove the clothing from the patient's uninjured side, then from the injured side.

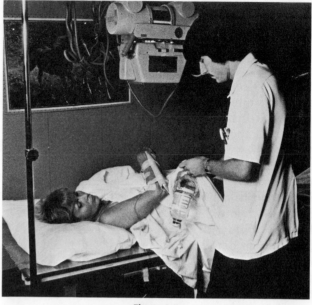

Figure 3-4

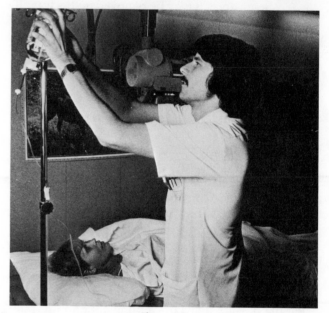

Figure 3-5

from the affected side. Next, gently lift the item over the patient's head. One person alone should not attempt to undress a disabled patient because this is apt to cause further injury or discomfort.

To remove trousers, loosen buckles and buttons and have the patient raise his buttocks. If he is unable to help, have two assistants raise the buttocks while another person slides the clothing off. Then remove the clothing over the legs and feet.

Fold the clothing and place it in a paper bag on which the patient's name has been printed. If the patient is accompanied by a relative or a friend, ask that person to keep the patient's clothing. If the patient is alone, the RT will be responsible for caring for the clothing.

When a patient's gown becomes wet or soiled in the radiology department, it is the RT's duty to change it. If a patient is allowed to remain in a wet or soiled gown his skin may become damaged or he may become chilled.

When changing the gown of a patient who has an injury or is paralyzed on one side, remove the gown from the uninjured side first. Then, with the

patient covered by the soiled gown, place the clean gown on the affected side, and then on the unaffected side. Pull the soiled gown from under the clean gown.

Frequently patients are taken to the radiology department with an intravenous infusion running. If the patient's gown must be changed, the clothing should be slipped off the unaffected side first. Then carefully slide the sleeve on the affected side over the intravenous tubing and catheter, then over the bottle of fluid. For this step, the bottle must be removed from the standard. When replacing a soiled gown with a clean one, first place the sleeve on the affected side over the bottle of fluid, then over the tubing and onto the arm with the venous catheter in place (Fig. 3-4). Rehang the bottle of fluid and complete the change (Fig. 3-5). When moving the arm of a patient who has an intravenous catheter in place, support the arm firmly so that the catheter does not become dislodged. Remember to keep the bottle of fluid above the infusion site, to prevent blood from flowing into the tubing.

Assisting Patients with Bedpan or Urinal

A patient may spend several hours in the radiology department; often he is not able to postpone urination or defecation. The patient may be embarrassed about making the required request, and will wait until the last possible moment to do so. When such a request is made, the RT should respond quickly and treat it in a matter-of-fact manner.

If possible, help the patient reach the lavatory near his examining room; this is the most desirable way to handle the situation. However, do not allow the patient to go to the toilet without assistance. Help him to put on his slippers or shoes, and wrap a draw sheet around him if no robe is available. Help him off the radiographic table or out of his wheelchair, and lead him to the lavatory. A patient may have been fasting, or may have been given drugs which make him very unsteady; therefore it is not safe to leave him unattended. If the patient can help himself in the lavatory, close the door and tell him that you will be just outside in case he needs you. Each lavatory should be equipped with an emergency call button, and the RT should explain its use to the patient. If there is no emergency call button, the RT should check on the patient at frequent intervals to be certain that his condition is stable.

After the patient has finished using the lavatory, help him wash his hands if he cannot do it

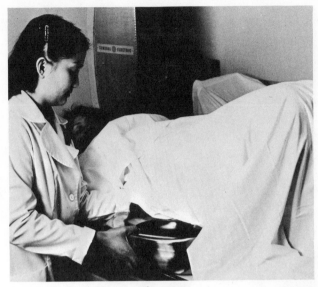

Figure 3-7

himself. Then accompany him back to the examination area. Cover the patient if necessary and make him comfortable. Return to the lavatory and make certain that it is clean.

The patient who is unable to get to the lavatory must be offered a bedpan or a urinal. In the radiology department, clean bedpans and urinals usually are stored in a specific place. Be certain that the bedpan or urinal that is to be used has been sterilized between uses.

There are two types of bedpans. The standard bedpan is made of metal or plastic and is approximately four inches high. It can be used by most patients. However, a patient may have a fracture or another disability that makes it impossible for him to use a pan of this height. For these patients the fracture pan is used. All radiology departments should make these pans available (Fig. 3-6).

Before assisting the patient, the RT must wash his hands and then obtain tissues and a bedpan with a cover. If the pan is cold, run warm water over it, then dry it. If possible, close the examining room door, or screen the patient to ensure privacy.

Always place a sheet over the patient while assisting him onto the bedpan. Approach the patient; remove the bedpan cover and place it at the end of the table. If the patient is able to move himself, ask him to raise his hips. Place the pan under the patient's hips (Fig. 3-7). Be sure he is covered with a sheet. If he is able to sit up, assist him to a sitting position. *Do not leave a patient sitting on a bedpan*—he is poorly balanced and may fall. If the RT cannot stay with the patient or the patient is not able to sit up, obtain two or three pillows and place them behind his shoulders and head so that he is comfortable (Fig. 3-8). Leave the

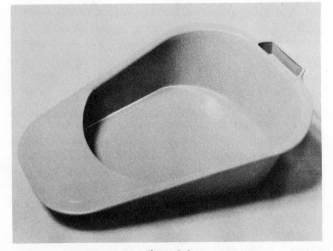

Figure 3-6

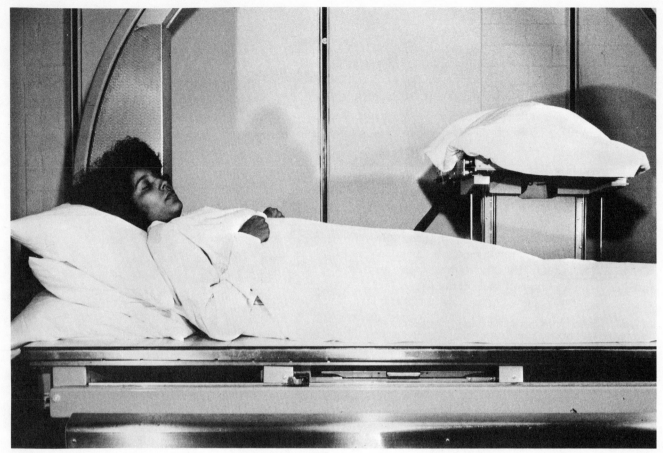

Figure 3-8

toilet tissue where he can reach it. Leave the patient alone, but remain nearby so that when he has finished you are on hand to assist him.

When the patient has finished using the bedpan, help him off the pan by having him lie back and raise his hips as you remove the pan. Cover the pan, empty it, and rinse it clean with cold water; then return it to the area where used equipment is placed.

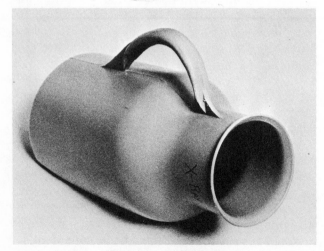

Figure 3-9. Male urinal.

Wash your hands and offer the patient a wet wash cloth or paper towel to wash his hands with and then a dry paper towel to dry them.

If a patient is unable to assist in getting himself on and off a bedpan, do not attempt to help him alone. Enlist the aid of another team member. Have that person stand at the opposite side of the table. With the assistance of the second RT, roll the patient to the distal side of the table. Place the pan against the patient's hips, then roll him to a supine position while holding the pan in place. Be certain that his hips are in good alignment on the pan. Place pillows under his shoulders and head and stay nearby. When he has finished using the pan, repeat the above procedure to remove him from the pan. If the patient is not able to clean the perineal area, the RT will have to assist him. Take several thicknesses of tissue and fold them into a pad to protect your hand. Wipe the patient's perineum from front to back, then drop the tissue in the pan; if necessary, repeat the procedure until the perineum is clean and dry. Cover the pan and empty it, then wash your hands as for heavy contamination.

If a patient has difficulty in moving or adjusting to the height of a regular bedpan, the same procedure may be followed using a fracture pan.

The Male Urinal

The male urinal is made of plastic or metal and is so shaped that it can be used by a patient who is supine, lying on his right or his left side, or in Fowler's position. The urinal may be offered to the male patient who is unable to get off the gurney or examining table to go to the lavatory (Fig. 3-9).

If the patient is able to help himself, simply hand him an aseptic urinal and allow him to use it, providing privacy whenever possible. When he has finished, remove the urinal, empty it, and rinse it with cold water; place it with the soiled supplies to be resterilized. Offer the patient a wash cloth to cleanse his hands. The RT must remember to wash his own hands also.

If a patient is unable to assist himself in using the urinal, the RT will position the urinal for him. Raise the cover sheet sufficiently to permit adequate visibility, but do not unduly expose the patient. Separate the patient's legs and put the urinal between them. Place the penis into the urinal far enough so that it does not slip out, and hold the urinal in place by the handle until the patient finishes voiding. Remove the urinal, empty it, replace it, and wash your hands.

Summary

When an outpatient arrives in the radiology department, it often is necessary that he undress entirely or partially for the radiologic procedure. The RT should always show the patient exactly where and how this is to be done in order to avoid uncertainty and embarrassment for the patient.

It is also the RT's responsibility to provide the patient with a safe place for his personal belongings. Remember that an item that may not seem valuable to the RT may be treasured by the patient. Every item that belongs to a patient must be treated as if it were of value.

If an outpatient cannot help himself undress and is not accompanied by someone to help him, the RT must offer assistance. This assistance should be given in a matter-of-fact manner so that the patient's privacy is not violated and he is spared embarrassment.

A patient who is totally disabled must be kept clean and dry while in the radiology department. It will be the RT's duty to change the patient's gown and covering if it becomes wet or soiled. This should be done in a prescribed way to ensure the patient's privacy, safety, and comfort.

Some examinations done in the radiology department are long and tedious. They often stimulate peristalsis and a need to defecate or urinate. Meeting these needs cannot be postponed. The RT must be prepared to assist the patient with a bedpan or urinal if necessary. This should be done in a way that assures the patient as much privacy as is possible. The patient should never be left unattended while on a bedpan, a gurney, or an x-ray table.

Patients are often in a weakened state due to illness or because they have fasted prior to the examination. They must be carefully attended when they are taken to a lavatory or a dressing area.

Bedpans and urinals should be used for only one patient and then returned to the central supply station for re-sterilization. The RT must always remember to use good medical aseptic techniques when assisting patients to dress or undress or to use bedpans and urinals. His hands must be washed before and after he attends each patient. All equipment must be clean before it is used.

See Appendix for pre-post test on Chapter 3.

Body Mechanics, Skin Care, and Moving of Patients

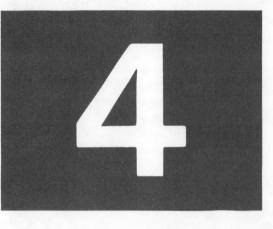

4

Goal of This Chapter

The RT student must learn how to move and lift patients in a manner that is safe for the patient and for himself, as well as how to protect the patient's skin from being damaged.

Objectives

When the student has completed this chapter, he will be able to:

1. Demonstrate, in a laboratory situation, the correct manner of moving and lifting patients to prevent injury to himself and the patient.
2. List four safety factors that must be considered when moving a patient.
3. Demonstrate, in the laboratory, the positioning of a patient to maintain good body alignment.
4. List three safety measures that must be taken when transferring a patient from the hospital ward to the radiology department and returning him to the ward.
5. List three situations in the radiology department that might result in damage to a patient's skin.
6. Demonstrate, in the laboratory, the correct method of moving a patient who is wearing a plaster cast.
7. List four possible signs of circulatory impairment that must be recognized by the RT.

Glossary

abrasion an area of the body surface denuded of skin or mucous membrane by some unusual or abnormal mechanical process

alignment having parts in proper relationship to each other

ambulation the act of walking

The RT, as a member of the health team, has the responsibility of protecting himself and his patients from injury in every way possible. Health workers often are injured while moving and lifting patients; yet almost all of these injuries can be prevented if the RT will practice good body mechanics at all times.

Patients are also the victims of injuries caused when they are improperly moved or lifted, and most of these injuries also can be prevented.

The RT must protect the patient's skin from injury, too. This is a problem particularly when a patient is unable to move himself. The RT must be aware of how skin damage may occur in order to take the precautions necessary to prevent it.

Body Mechanics

Constant abuse to one's spine from lifting patients is the leading cause of injuries to health care personnel in all health care institutions. The RT will be less fatigued and will avoid injury to himself if he follows the rules of good body mechanics. These rules are based on the laws of gravity.

Gravity is a force which pulls objects toward the center of the earth. Any movement made requires an expenditure of energy to overcome the force of gravity. When an object is balanced, it is firm and stable. If it is off balance, it will fall because of the pull of gravity. The center of gravity is the point at which the mass of any body is centered. When a person is standing, the center of gravity is the center of his

Glossary cont.

body mechanics   the efficient use of the body as a machine

bony prominence   an area where a bone protrudes and is covered by only a thin layer of skin; e.g., elbows, scapulae, knees, coccyx

circulation   movement in a regular or circuitous course, as the movement of the blood through the heart and blood vessels

decubitus ulcer   an area of inflamed and dead tissue caused by prolonged pressure; often found when patients are allowed to lie in one position for too long a period of time on a bed or hard surface

gravity   the quality of having weight, the gravitational attraction of the mass to the center of its universe

lateral   pertaining to a side

posture   the position of the body, or the way in which it is held

prone   lying face down

supine   lying face up

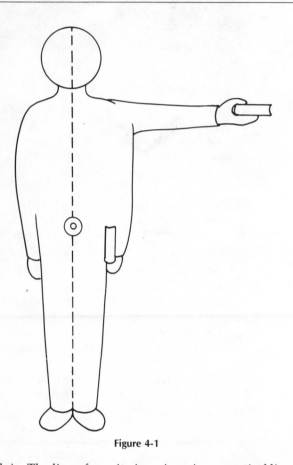

Figure 4-1

pelvis. The line of gravity is an imaginary vertical line that passes through the center of gravity. The base of support for a person standing is his two feet (Fig. 4-1).

Good body mechanics requires good posture. Good posture means that the body is in proper alignment with all parts in balance—this permits the musculoskeletal system (the bones and joints) to work at maximum efficiency. Good posture also aids other body systems. For instance, if the chest is held up and out (musculoskeletal system), the lungs can work with greater efficiency (respiratory system).

General rules for correct upright posture are:
1. Stand with the feet parallel and at right angles to the lower legs. Feet should be parted about four to eight inches. Keep body weight equally distributed on both feet.
2. Keep the knees slightly bent because this acts as a "shock absorber" for the body.
3. Keep the buttocks in and the abdomen up and in. This prevents strain on the back and abdominal muscles.
4. The chest should be held up and slightly forward with the waist extended. This allows the lungs to expand properly and fill to the greatest possible capacity.
5. The head should be held erect with the chin held in. This puts, the spine in proper alignment and there is no curve in the neck.

When moving and lifting objects or patients, the RT should always remember to protect himself by keeping the body's line of balance close to the center of gravity, which is at or just below the waistline. When picking an object up from the floor, bend the knees and lower your body. Do not bend from the waist. The biceps muscles are the strongest arm muscles and are effective in pulling; therefore, pull weight, do not push it (Fig. 4-2).

When a patient must be lifted, balance the load over both feet. Hold the load close to your body, bend your knees, and set your spine to support the load. Use your arm and leg muscles to lift. The spine must always be protected. Instead of twisting your body to move with a load, change foot positions. Always keep your body balanced over your two feet, which are spread to provide a firm base of support. Make certain that the floor area where the work is being done is clear of all objects.

Moving and Transferring Patients

The RT will occasionally be called upon to transfer a patient to or from a hospital ward, or he may have to direct a porter to do this. Certain precautions must be taken when this is to be done to make sure the *right* patient is transported at the *right* time, for the *right* procedure, and in as safe a manner as is possible.

After being informed of the patient's name and room number, and the radiographic procedure to be done, the RT or porter should go to the nurse's station on the ward where the patient is in residence. The nurse in charge should be told who is wanted and for what procedure. She will hand the RT that patient's chart. Specific precautions to be followed for the patient should be requested at this time. Then the RT proceeds to the patient's room, greets him, and checks his identifying name band with his chart. When it is certain that he is the correct patient, proceed with the transfer.

When returning a patient to his hospital room, stop at the nurse's station, return the chart to the desk, and inform the ward personnel that the patient is being returned to his room. The ward staff must always be notified before the patient is returned to his room. If help is needed to return the patient to his bed, request it at this time. The RT or a porter must never attempt to transfer a patient from a gurney to a hospital bed without assistance.

Before the RT begins to move a patient, he must assess the patient's ability to aid in the process. He must also decide how the patient can best be transferred—by gurney or wheelchair. If there is any question about what the patient can do for himself, the nurse or person in charge of the ward should be consulted. In assessing the patient's abilities, the RT has to consider such problems as the following:

1. The patient's condition: how well, or how poorly, is he functioning?
2. The patient's mobility: are his motions restricted in any way?
3. The patient's strength and endurance: will he become fatigued and be unable to complete the transfer without assistance?
4. The patient's ability to maintain his balance: can he sit or stand and maintain this position?
5. The patient's ability to understand what is expected of him during the transfer: is he responsive and alert?
6. The patient's acceptance of the move: does he fear or resent the transfer? Will the transfer increase his pain or does he feel that it is unnecessary?

After the RT has completed his assessment and has judged the patient's capabilities, he must decide how the patient can best be moved and how much help will be needed to safely execute the move. A patient must not be moved without adequate assistance; to do so may cause injury to the patient or to the RT. Rules to remember when moving patients are the following:

1. Give only the assistance that the patient needs for comfort and safety.

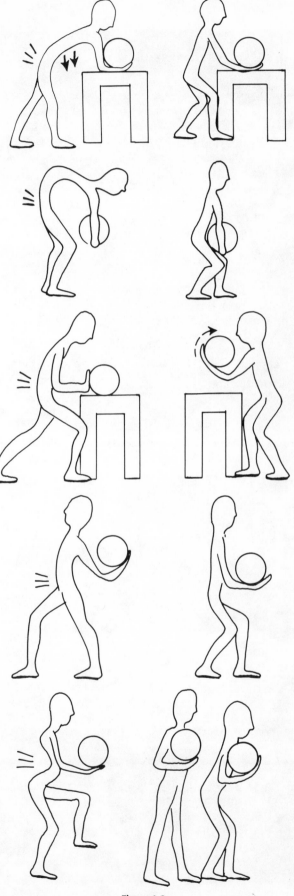

Figure 4-2

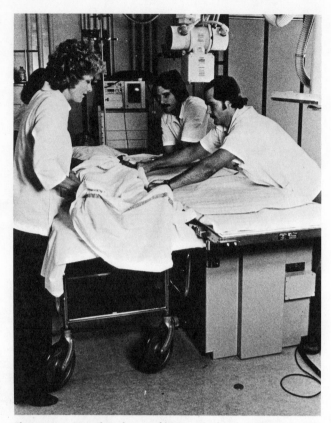

Figure 4-3. Move in unison, making certain that the patient's head is supported during the transfer.

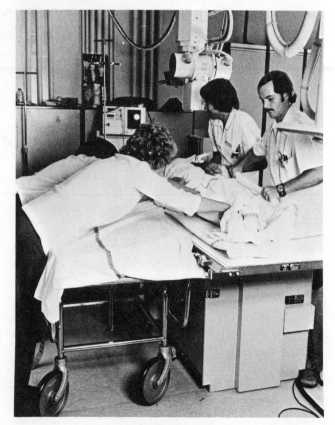

Figure 4-4

2. Always transfer a patient across the shortest distance.
3. Lock all wheels on beds, gurneys, and wheelchairs.
4. Generally it is better to move a patient toward his strong side while the RT assists at his weak side.
5. The patient should wear shoes for standing transfers, but slippery bedroom slippers should not be worn.
6. The patient must be informed of the plan of the move, and his help encouraged.
7. The patient should be given short, simple commands and the RT must help the patient carry them out.

Methods of Transfer

There are essentially three ways of transferring patients: by gurney, by wheelchair, and by patient ambulation. When a patient is moved from a gurney to a radiographic table, or the reverse, great care must be exercised to prevent injury. If the patient is unconscious or unable to cooperate in the move, his spine, head, and extremities must be well supported. One convenient way to do this is to place a sheet under him and use this sheet to slide him from one surface to another. If the patient is an adult, three or four people should participate in the maneuver. One person stands at the patient's head to guide and support it during the move; another should be at the side of the surface to which the patient will be moved; and the third person should be at the side of the surface on which the patient is lying. If there are four people, two may stand at each side. The sheet is rolled at the side of the patient so that the RT can easily grasp it in his hands close to the patient's body. The team should be in agreement (usually by a count of 1, 2, 3) about when the move will begin. In unison, they transfer the patient to the other surface (Figs. 4-3 and 4-4).

If the radiographic table is a stationary cradle type, extra padding should be placed over the metal parts at the table's edge to protect the patient from being bruised as he is moved (Fig. 4-5). Some cradle tables have a floating top. In this case, the top should be moved forward close to the edge of the gurney. Conscious patients should be cautioned that the center part of these tables is lower than the surface so that they are not frightened when lowered into it.

Tube housings above radiographic tables should be moved out of the way when patients are being moved to protect both patients and RTs from bumping into them in the moving process. A stationary unit such as a fluoroscopic unit must be considered when moving patients. To avoid bumping the

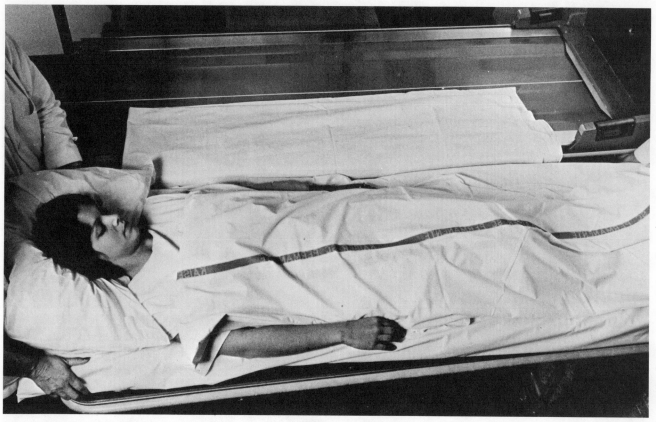

Figure 4-5

unit, the patient should be warned not to sit up, and the RT must also be careful not to injure himself by bumping stationary units.

A three-carrier lift can be used to move a patient from one place to another. This lift, if properly performed, can be accomplished without injury to patient or technologist. Begin by sliding the patient to the edge of the area from which he is to be lifted. Have the gurney at a right angle at the end of the radiographic table with the wheel locked. All three persons who are going to lift the patient then go to that side of the table; one stands at the patient's head and neck, one at the buttocks, and one at the legs and ankles (Fig. 4-6). Cross the patient's arms over his chest. The lifters all place their bodies against the area on which the patient is lying and place their arms under the part of the patient that they are going to lift.

At the signal the movers roll the patient off the table and onto their chests (Fig. 4-7). All three pivot and place the patient on the area to which he is being moved (Fig. 4-8).

If a patient must be moved from a bed or radiographic table to a wheelchair, or the reverse, he must be helped. The RT must never allow a patient to get off a table or into a wheelchair without some assistance. The patient is often not as strong as he believes himself to be. The sudden movement may

cause dizziness and the patient may fall. If the patient has been in a supine position and is to be helped to a sitting position, the RT should have him turn to his side with his knees flexed (Fig. 4-9). Then the RT may place himself in front of the patient with one arm around the shoulders of the patient and the other arm at the knees. He may then help the patient to sit at the edge of the table. Before assisting the patient to stand, allow him to sit for a moment and regain his sense of balance (Fig. 4-10). Then, if the patient needs further assistance, the RT may place himself in front of the patient, bend his knees, flex one knee against the table, place his arms at the patient's sides, and assist him to stand (Fig. 4-11). If the patient needs only minimal assistance, the RT may stand at the patient's side and take his arm to assist him off the table.

The RT should never allow a patient to step down from a radiographic table if it is high without providing a secure stepping stool for him to step onto before he steps to the floor. The RT should always stay at the patient's side to assist him.

If the patient is to be seated in a wheelchair, have the chair facing him. It must be close enough so that the patient can be seated in the wheelchair with one pivot. Have the foot supports of the chair up and the wheels locked (Fig. 4-12). The RT should stand in front of the patient, spread his feet for a broad base of

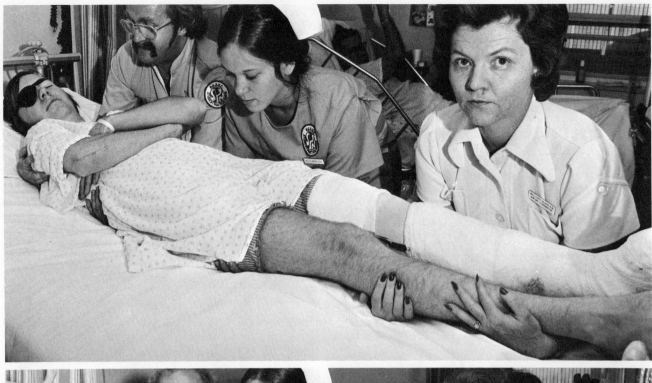

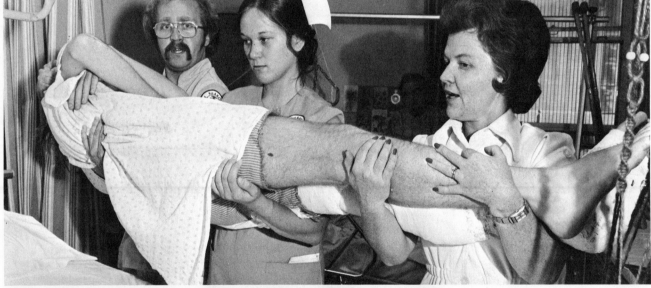

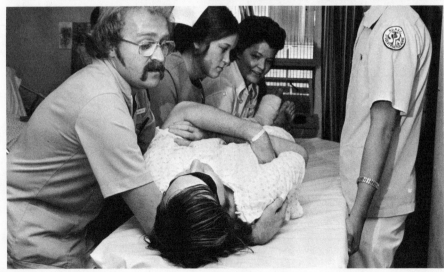

Figures 4-6 through 4-8 are from LuVerne Wolff Lewis, *Fundamental Skills in Patient Care* (Philadelphia, J. B. Lippincott Company, 1976), pp. 246–48.

support, flex his knees, support the patient at his sides, pivot with the patient, and seat him in the chair (Fig. 4-13). The foot rests on the wheelchair should then be put up and the wheels unlocked.

The patient must be kept covered as much as possible during any moving or transferring procedures. A patient should never be transferred by gurney or wheelchair without being covered with a sheet or bath blanket. When a patient is placed on the radiographic table, he must be covered with a protective sheet. He must not be allowed to become chilled if it is at all possible to prevent this. A confused, disoriented, or unconscious patient or a child must never be left alone on a radiographic table or a gurney. If the patient is not dependable and is in a wheelchair he should be observed carefully. A soft restraint belt should be placed over all patients who are left on gurneys. If the gurney has side rails, they should be up (Fig. 4-14).

Positioning Patients

Patients must be kept positioned so that their bodies are in good alignment on the radiographic table. If the patient is in a supine position, he must be placed with his head, neck, and spine in a straight line. The arms and legs should be parallel to his body and hips, and the knees and feet should be straight when radiographic exposures are not being made (Fig. 4-15).

To move a helpless patient to a lateral position for an examination, move him to the side of the table to which his back will be turned. Obtain help to move the patient if necessary. First the patient's head, neck, and shoulders should be moved. The RT then places his hands and lower arms under the patient's hips and moves the trunk and hips. The process is repeated to move the legs. If there is a pull sheet under the patient, he can be moved with the pull sheet.

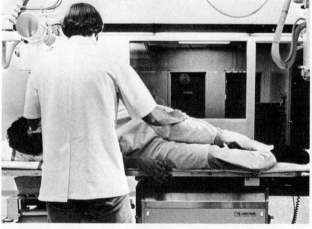

Figure 4-9

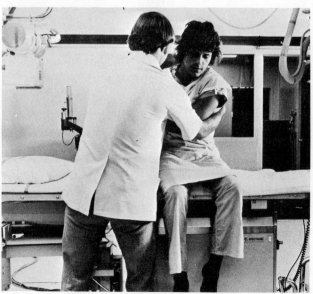

Figure 4-10

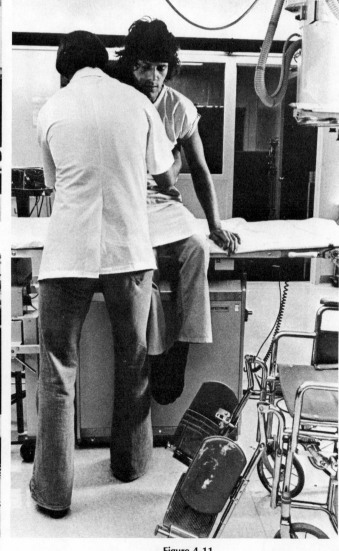

Figure 4-11

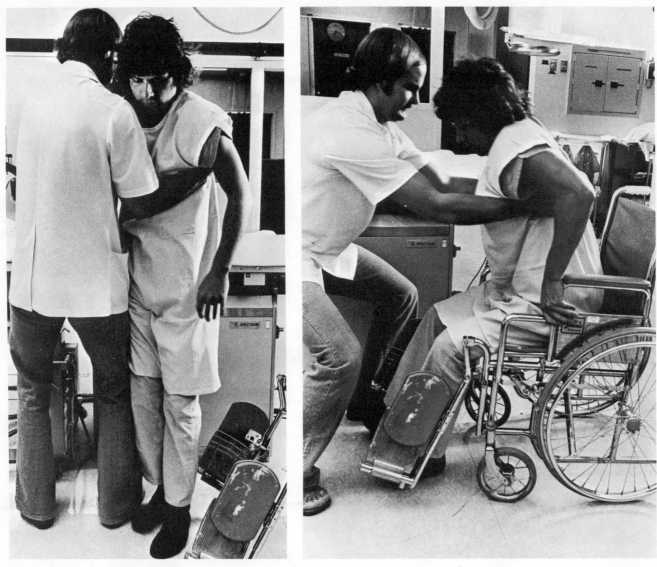

Figure 4-12

Figure 4-13

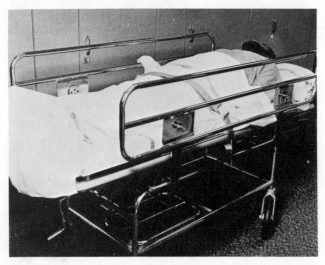

Figure 4-14

When the patient is lying on his side, the RT must be certain that his arm is not under him. Keep the patient's neck, head, and back in a straight line. Flex the upper leg so that it is not resting on the lower leg. Use pillows or bolsters to support the patient if this is possible (Fig. 4-16).

If the patient must be in a prone position, first turn him to his side and then continue to roll him until he is lying on his stomach. Turn the patient's head to one side. His body should be straight, with the arms parallel to the body and the legs straight (Fig. 4-17).

When moving a patient to an unnatural position for a radiographic exposure, leave him in that position for only the length of time necessary and then return him to a position in which his body is in good alignment.

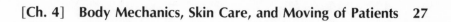

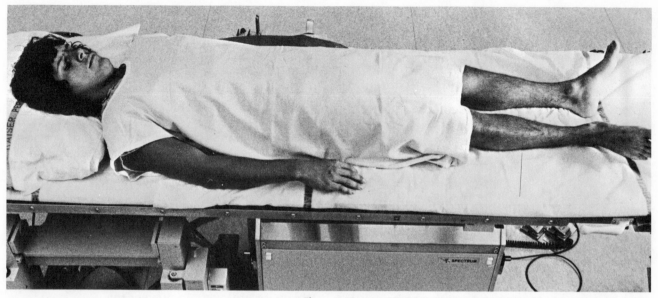

Figure 4-15

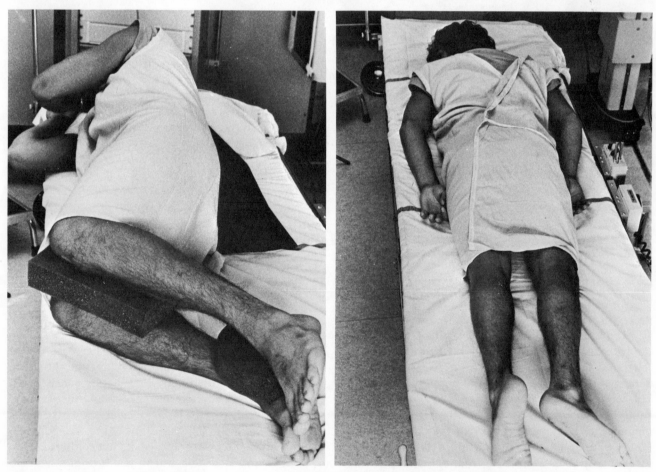

Figure 4-16

Figure 4-17

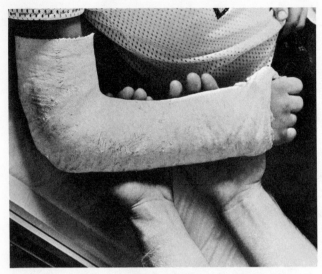

Figure 4-18

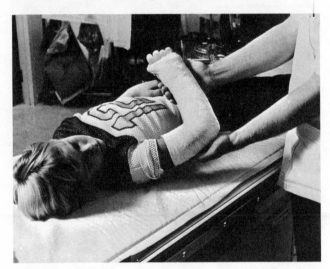

Figure 4-19

Skin Care

The RT will have to assume responsibility for protecting the patient's skin when he is in the radiology department. The radiographic table is a hard and unprotected surface, and if a patient must spend a relatively long period of time on it, the skin may be damaged due to pressure on the bony prominences. The weight of the body causes blood vessels to become constricted. In a very short time irreparable damage can be done, especially if the patient is old, poorly nourished, or in an unhealthy state. The areas most susceptible to pressure, redness, and eventual breakdown if not cared for are the scapulae, the sacrum, the trochanters, the knees, and the heels of the feet. A decubitus ulcer, or bed sore, can begin to form in two hours and, once started, is difficult to cure.

Heat, perspiration, urine, and feces can further aggravate skin that is mottled and reddened.

The RT should help a patient who is on a gurney or radiographic table for long periods of time to change his position or should change it for him if he is unable to do this. Pressure should be kept off hips, knees, and heels. This can be done by placing a pillow or a soft blanket under the patient or turning him to a different position whenever possible. In the usual hospital situation this is done routinely every two hours, but if a patient is lying on a hard surface it should be done every thirty minutes. If the patient is perspiring profusely or is incontinent of urine or feces, the RT should make certain that the patient is kept clean and dry.

Skin abrasions can occur if the patient is moved across the examining table too quickly or without enough help. Once the skin has been abraded, the danger of a decubitus ulcer is far greater. The RT should move patients on the radiographic table with great care to prevent this.

Cast Care

Patients will often arrive at the radiology department in a plaster cast of some sort. A fresh cast that is still damp can be compressed and the compression may produce pressure on the patient's skin. A cast can also cause circulatory impairment.

When moving a patient who has a newly applied plaster cast that is still wet, the RT should handle the cast with his hands open to create a flat surface. Avoid grasping a wet cast with the fingers because this produces indentations (Fig. 4-18). Support the cast when the patient is moving. If the cast is on an extremity, move the extremity for the patient as a whole unit, supporting the joint (Fig. 4-19). To position a patient who is in a cast, have pillows or sandbags on hand so that the cast can be well supported. If a cast is allowed to put pressure on the patient's skin in any area, it will cause impairment of circulation.

A patient who is in a plaster cast in the radiology department for any length of time should be checked for signs of impaired circulation every fifteen minutes. A cast applied to an arm may cause circulatory disturbance in the hand, a leg or body cast, in the feet, toes, or lower leg. The signs of impaired circulation that the RT may detect easily are coldness, complaint of fingers or toes burning and tingling, swelling, color changes (to pale or bluish color), and numbness or inability to move fingers or toes. If a patient complains of any of these symptoms or the RT can see or feel any of these changes, he should change the patient's position and notify the radiologist immediately.

Summary

The RT must practice good body mechanics in his work. Good body mechanics begins with good posture. When moving and lifting objects or patients, he must work close to his load and maintain a firm base of support by having his feet slightly spread and his knees flexed. Never twist the body or bend at the waist when lifting a heavy load. Weight should be pulled, not pushed. Arm and leg muscles, not the spine, should be used for lifting.

The three ways of moving patients are by gurney, wheelchair, and patient ambulation. When moving and lifting patients, the RT must assess the patient and solve potential problems before beginning the move. The plan of moving the patient should be explained to him and his help should be enlisted before beginning. The RT must always notify the ward personnel when he is taking a patient to and from his room in the hospital.

When a patient is on the radiographic table or on a gurney in the radiology department, his body must be in good alignment. If the patient must be moved to a particular position for an examination, good body alignment must be restored as quickly as possible.

The patient's skin can become damaged while he is in the radiology department. The RT must protect the patient from this by keeping his weight off the bony prominences of the body with frequent changes of position. There must not be pressure on any part for too long. The patient's skin should also be kept clean and dry to reduce possible skin irritation. Precautions should be taken to prevent skin abrasions when moving patients.

Plaster casts must be properly cared for, and the patient's extremities must be observed for circulatory impairment which may be caused by pressure of the cast on the skin. The symptoms of circulatory impairment are coldness, swelling, burning, tingling, color changes in the skin, and inability to move fingers or toes. The RT must change the patient's position if these symptoms occur and must report them to the radiologist immediately.

See Appendix for pre-post test on Chapter 4.

Vital Signs and Oxygen Administration

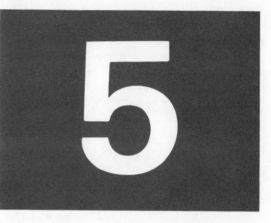

Goal of This Chapter

The RT student must be able to monitor vital signs accurately and be prepared to assist with the administration of oxygen.

Objectives

When the student has completed this chapter, he will be able to:

1. Correctly read a clinical thermometer as demonstrated in the laboratory.
2. Accurately monitor the pulse rate at five major arteries of the human body, as demonstrated in the laboratory.
3. Demonstrate in a laboratory setting the ability to monitor respirations.
4. Correctly monitor blood pressure in the laboratory setting.
5. List the rates of pulse, respiration, and blood pressure that are considered within normal limits for an adult male or female.
6. List the precautions the RT must take when oxygen is being administered in a patient's room or in the radiology department.

Glossary

anterior   situated in front of or in the forward part of an organ

apex   the point of greatest activity or greatest response to stimulation

axillary   pertaining to the axilla, a small pyramid shaped space between the upper lateral chest and the medial side of the arm

expiration   the act of exhaling or expelling air from the lungs

fever   elevation of body temperature above normal due to some physical change in the body

Accurate assessment of the patient's physical condition includes assessment of vital signs, which means temperature, pulse, respiration, and blood pressure. The RT must learn where and how to measure each vital sign, so that if he needs this assessment skill in an emergency situation he will be able to use it.

Oxygen administration is necessary occasionally in the radiology department and frequently in hospital rooms. If oxygen is administered in the radiology department, the RT will be expected to assist in its administration. Patients who are receiving oxygen therapy in their hospital room may be unable to leave their room to go to the radiology department for necessary radiographic exposures. In these instances, the RT will be required to make radiographic exposures with a portable machine at the bedside. Because oxygen is a potentially volatile substance, certain precautions must be taken when using radiographic equipment in this situation. The RT should also be acquainted with the various methods of oxygen administration.

Temperature

Body temperature must remain stable in order for the body's cellular function and enzymatic activity to remain efficient. Body temperature is a physiologic balance between heat produced in the tissues and the external environment and heat lost to the environment. When a patient's body temperature is elevated, we say that he has a *fever*, which indicates a disturbance in the heat-regulating center.

Glossary cont.

inspiration the act of drawing air into the lungs

oral by mouth

sphygmomanometer an instrument used for measuring blood pressure in the arteries

sternum a longitudinal plate of bone forming the middle of the anterior wall of the thorax and joining above with the clavicles and along the sides with the cartilages

stethoscope an instrument of various form, size, and material used for listening indirectly to body sounds

volatile explosive

Both normal and abnormal conditions of the body can produce changes in body temperature. Time of day, age, weight, physical exercise, disease, and injury are some of the factors that might influence body temperature.

A body temperature of 37° Celsius or 98.6° Fahrenheit is considered to be average or normal. A variation of one degree above or below average is not considered abnormal; if a patient's temperature is 36 or 38° Celsius (C) or 97.6 or 99° Fahrenheit (F), the reading would be considered within normal limits.

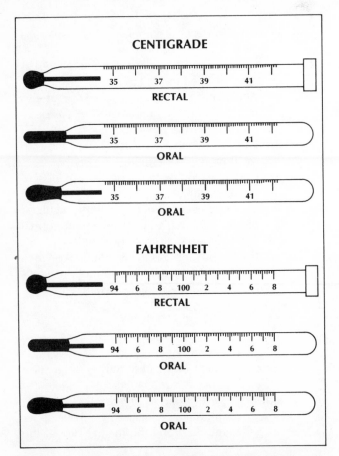

Figure 5-1. Glass clinical thermometers. Top: these three are calibrated to measure degrees in the centigrade scale; bottom: these three measure in the Fahrenheit scale. The thermometers with blunt bulbs are rectal thermometers. From LuVerne Wolff Lewis, *Fundamental Skills in Patient Care* (Philadelphia: J. B. Lippincott Company, 1976), p. 116.

There are three areas of the body in which temperature can be measured, and the reading may vary depending on where temperature is measured. Therefore the place where the temperature is taken must be specified when reporting the reading. Oral temperature is taken in the mouth, under the tongue; the average temperature reading here is 37° C (98.6° F). Axillary temperature is taken in the axilla or armpit; the average temperature reading here is 36.7° C (97.6° F). Rectal temperature is taken in the rectum; the average reading here is 38° C (99.6° F).

The RT must be certain that the thermometer used to measure a patient's temperature has been properly sterilized. The thermometer must never be wiped clean and re-used, but must be sterilized between uses. When measuring an oral temperature, obtain an oral thermometer which has an elongated tip. Shake the thermometer down to a mercury reading of 96° F or 35° C. Wash your hands, approach the patient, and place the thermometer under his tongue. Have the patient close his lips over the tip of the thermometer and leave it in place for from three to five minutes. Then remove it, wipe it with a tissue, and read it.

When reading a thermometer, hold it at eye level by the blunt end and move it until the mercury column can be seen. Observe where on the marked scale the mercury stops; this is the temperature to be recorded. Each long line on the thermometer represents one full degree of body temperature and is numbered. The short lines each represent two-tenths of one degree of body temperature, and these lines are not numbered. After the thermometer has been read, place it with the soiled thermometers. Wash your hands.

When it is necessary to take an axillary temperature, an oral thermometer may be used. Wash your hands and shake the thermometer down. Dry the patient's armpit with a dry paper towel or a dry wash cloth. Lift the patient's arm and place the thermometer in the armpit. Place the arm down tightly over the thermometer with the arm crossed over the chest. Leave the thermometer in place for five minutes. Then remove it, read it, wipe it, and put it in its proper place.

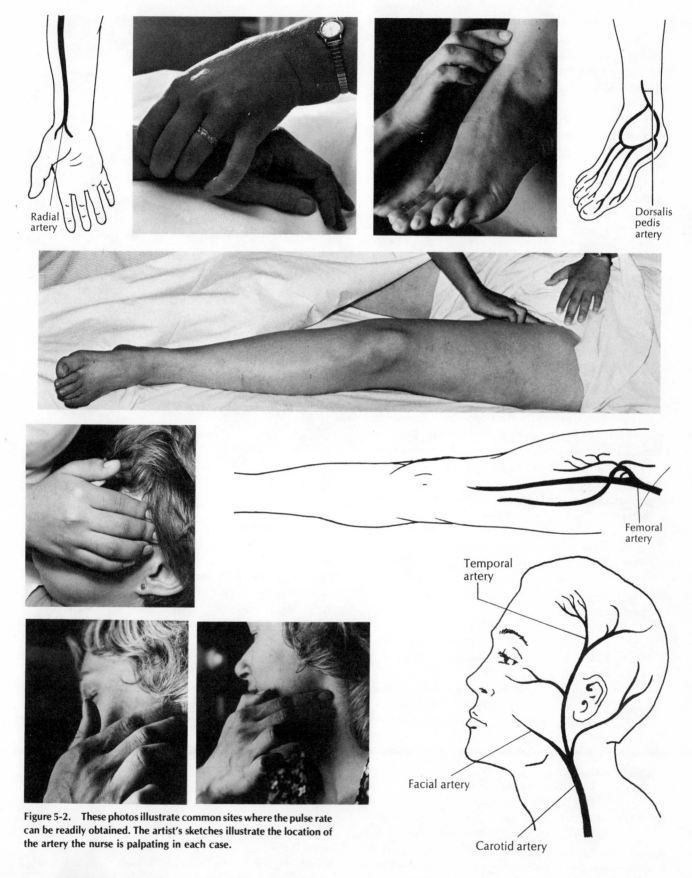

Figure 5-2. These photos illustrate common sites where the pulse rate can be readily obtained. The artist's sketches illustrate the location of the artery the nurse is palpating in each case.

To take a rectal temperature, a thermometer with a blunt tip must be used. Do not use an oral thermometer to take a rectal temperature. Wash your hands. Have the patient turn on his side, and expose only as much as is necessary for clearly viewing the rectal area. Lubricate the tip of the thermometer with a lubricating jelly. Insert it into the rectum about one and one-half inches. Hold the thermometer in place for two to three minutes. Do not leave a patient who has a rectal thermometer in place. The thermometer must be held. When enough time has passed, remove the thermometer. Return the patient to a comfortable position and wipe the thermometer with a tissue. Read it and place it with the soiled rectal thermometers. Wash your hands.

Temperature readings are recorded in the hospital as follows: a rectal temperature of 99.6 degrees is written as 99.6 R.; an oral temperature of 98.6° is written as 98.6 O.; an axillary temperature of 97.6° is written as 97.6 Ax. (Fig. 5-1).

Pulse

As the heart beats, blood is sent through the arteries, and this results in a throb or a pulsation of the artery. At areas of the body where the arteries are superficial, the pulse can be felt by holding the artery beneath the skin against a solid surface such as bone. The pulse can be felt most easily at the following six places in the body:

1. The radial pulse—over the radial artery at the wrist, at the base of the thumb.
2. The temporal pulse—over the temporal artery in front of the ear.
3. The carotid pulse—over the carotid artery at the front of the neck.
4. The femoral pulse—over the femoral artery in the groin.
5. The apical pulse—over the apex of the heart; this pulse is heard with a stethoscope and not felt.
6. The pedal pulse—over the dorsal pedal artery at the arch of the foot (Fig. 5-2).

Usually the pulse rate is rapid if the blood pressure is low and slower if the blood pressure is high. The patient who is losing blood has an unusually high pulse rate and a low blood pressure. The average pulse rate in an adult male or female is 70 to 80 beats per minute in a state of rest. The average rate in an infant is 115 to 130 beats per minute, in an older person, 56 to 60 beats per minute. Excitement, fever, hemorrhage, and exercise cause the pulse rate to rise.

When the pulse rate is being monitored, it is important to note the strength and regularity of the beat as well as the number of beats per minute. To take a pulse one needs a watch with a second hand and a

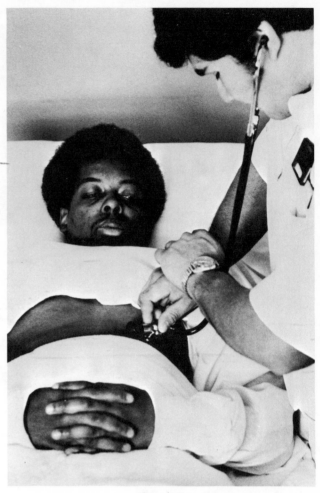

Figure 5-3

pad and pencil to record the count. To monitor the apical pulse, a stethoscope is necessary along with an alcohol sponge for wiping the earpieces of the stethoscope. To monitor the radial, femoral, carotid, and temporal pulse, wash your hands, approach the patient, and place your index finger and middle finger lightly and flatly over the artery. Do not press too hard or your fingers will compress the artery, and the beat will not be felt. When the throbbing of the artery is felt, count the throbs for one minute. Do not use the thumb when counting pulse rate because it too has a pulse, which may be mistaken for the patient's pulse rate.

To monitor the apical pulse, wash your hands, wipe the earpiece of the stethoscope, approach the patient, and place him in a comfortable sitting or supine position. Lift his clothing so as to expose the lower chest area. Place the bell of the stethoscope to the left of the sternum and between the fifth and sixth ribs. If the beat cannot be heard, move the stethoscope slightly in every direction until it can be heard. Count the beats for one minute. Remove the stethoscope, wipe the ear pieces and the bell with an alcohol pad, cover the patient, wash your hands, and record the pulse (Fig. 5-3).

Respiration

The function of the respiratory system is to exchange oxygen and carbon dioxide between the external environment and the blood circulating in the body. Oxygen is taken into the lungs during inspiration. It enters the arterioles, then is carried to the arteries, thence to the heart from which it is pumped. Thus oxygen is carried to all parts of the body. The blood is returned to the heart through the veins, and carbon dioxide is exhaled from the lungs during expiration.

The average rate of respiration in an adult male or female is sixteen to twenty per minute, and in an infant, thirty to fifty per minute. Respirations of less than ten per minute in an adult may result in cyanosis, apprehension, restlessness, and change of level of consciousness because the supply of oxygen is inadequate.

Respirations may be described as rapid, shallow, labored, regular, or irregular. When respirations are counted the quality as well as the number should be noted. Each inspiration-expiration counts as one respiratory beat.

The patient should be in a sitting or supine position when respirations are being counted. He

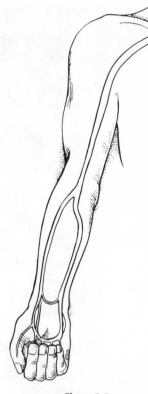

Figure 5-5

should be in a quiet state and should remain unaware that respirations are being assessed. When a patient suspects that his respirations are being observed, he may consciously or unconsciously cause the rate and quality to change. The most convenient time to count respirations is immediately following the pulse count. The technologist may appear to be continuing to count the pulse rate but may be observing the respirations instead. The respirations are counted by observing and counting the rise and fall of the patient's chest.

Blood Pressure

Blood pressure is the pressure exerted by the blood on the wall of a vessel. The instrument used to measure blood pressure is called a sphygmomanometer (Fig. 5-4). Two numbers are read and recorded when reporting blood pressure. These are the systolic pressure, which is the highest point that is reached by the contractions of the heart, and the diastolic pressure, which is the lowest point to which the pressure drops between contractions.

Blood pressure readings vary with age, sex, physical development, and health status. The normal systolic pressure in adult males and females ranges from 110 to 140 millimeters of mercury, the normal diastolic, from 60 to 90 millimeters of mercury (mm.

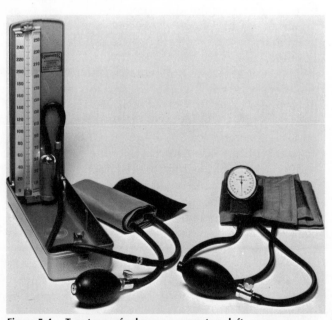

Figure 5-4. Two types of sphygmomanometers: left, a mercury manometer; right, an aneroid manometer. The cuffs are self-securing. There are several varieties of aneroid manometers. From LuVerne Wolff Lewis, *Fundamental Skills in Patient Care* (Philadelphia: J. B. Lippincott Company, 1976), p. 132.

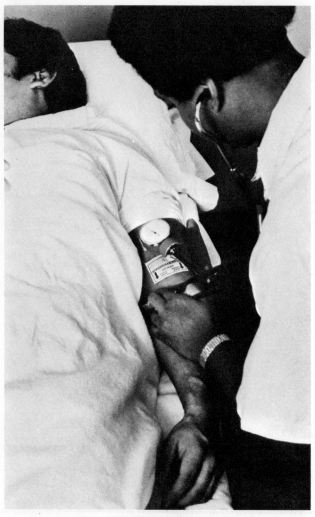

Figure 5-6

Hg). Blood pressure is measured by placing the sphygmomanometer cuff around the patient's upper arm above the elbow and placing the bell of a stethoscope over the brachial artery, located at the center of the anterior elbow area. This artery is readily identified by its pulsations (Fig. 5-5).

Place the gauge of the sphygmomanometer on a flat surface so that it can be read easily. The patient should be in a sitting or lying position. Secure the cuff of the sphygmomanometer so that it will not work loose. Place the earpieces of the stethoscope in your ears, tighten the thumbscrew on the air bulb, and pump the air bulb until it reaches 180 mm. Hg or until you no longer hear the pulse beat. Open the valve slowly and allow the mercury to fall. Listen carefully for the pulse beat sound to begin and take the reading where it is heard. This first reading will be the systolic reading. Continue to listen until the pulsation becomes soft or quiet. Note where the sound changes from loud to very soft. This is the diastolic reading.

Blood pressure is recorded in the following manner: if the systolic reading is 120 and the diastolic reading is 80 it is written 120/80 (Fig. 5-6).

Oxygen Therapy

Human beings must have oxygen to live, and oxygen cannot be stored in the body. When anoxia (inadequate oxygen supply) is present, oxygen therapy is usually begun. This treatment must be ordered by a physician, and the order will specify the method of administration and the concentration preferred. The RT must be acquainted with the methods of oxygen administration available in the radiology department in which he is employed, as well as the means used in other parts of the hospital. In his own department he may be called upon to assist with oxygen administration in an emergency situation; he will observe oxygen being administered in other sections of the hospital. Oxygen supports combustion; therefore, care must be taken to prevent sparks or flames where oxygen is being used. Since radiographic equipment may produce such a spark, the RT must take precautions when his equipment is to be used in the presence of pure oxygen.

There are many types of illness that may require oxygen therapy. For example, in lung diseases, oxygen is added to air to be inhaled by the patient, to ensure sufficient oxygen in his blood. In some heart conditions, the circulation of blood through the lungs may be impaired; an increased intake of oxygen will help to relieve the anoxia. When strict bed rest is an important part of therapy, oxygen may be administered so that the patient will expend as little energy as possible.

Often seriously ill patients who require oxygen therapy may not be able to come to the radiology department, and the RT will be required to take radiographic exposures in the patient's room with a portable machine. In these situations, the RT must consult with the nurse in charge of the patient's care and be advised of the limits placed upon the patient's activity. When a patient is receiving continuous oxygen, the RT must be certain that all of the preparations that need to be made before making an exposure are complete. Then he must have an assistant turn off the oxygen for only a brief moment while taking the exposure. With new radiographic equipment, it may not be necessary to discontinue the oxygen. The RT must familiarize himself with the rules of the hospital in this case.

During oxygen therapy, oxygen is delivered to the respiratory tract under pressure by artificial means. If the oxygen is not humidified, the mucous

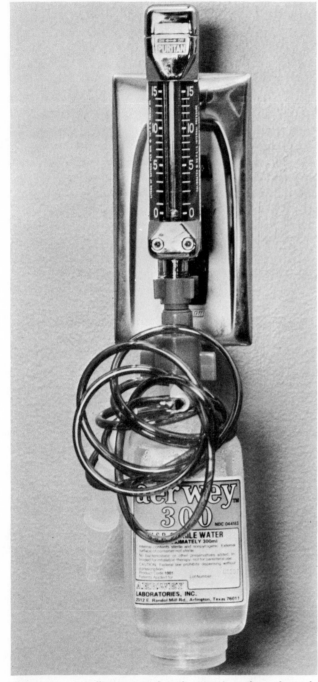

Figure 5-7.   A wall oxygen outlet. The container above the outlet contains sterile water for humidifying the oxygen. The flowmeter is located below the container.

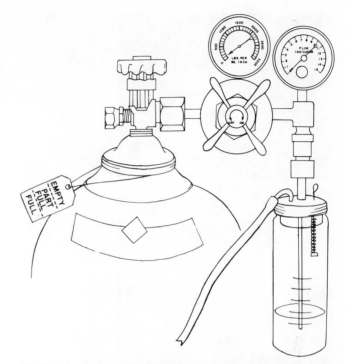

Figure 5-8.   Oxygen tank. The regulator valve on top of the tank allows the oxygen to flow out of the tank. The valve to the right of the tank regulates the flow. The gauge on the left indicates the amount of oxygen present in the tank; the one on the right indicates the rate of flow. The container to the right of the tank is a humidifier. From LuVerne Wolff Lewis, *Fundamental Skills in Patient Care* (Philadelphia: J. B. Lippincott Company, 1976), p. 404.

the radiology department. Tapping the wall outlets makes it readily available. Oxygen supplied in this fashion comes from a central source through pipes at 60 to 80 pounds of pressure per square inch. The average rate at which it is administered to patients is 4 to 5 liters per minute. A flow meter is attached to each wall outlet to regulate flow (Fig. 5-7).

In some radiology departments oxygen is not piped in and available through wall outlets, but is compressed and dispensed in tanks. A large full tank contains 2000 pounds per square inch of pressure. These tanks have two regulator valves, one of which indicates how much oxygen is in the tank and the other, the rate of flow. If the RT must use this type of system, care must be taken not to allow the tank to fall or the regulator to become cracked (Fig. 5-8).

There are several methods of administering oxygen to a patient: nasal cannula, face mask, nasal catheter, and tent. Of these, the cannula, a disposable plastic device which is held in place by means of a plastic strap placed around the patient's head, is one of the simplest methods and is used frequently to administer a high concentration of oxygen (Fig. 5-9).

A face mask covers the mouth and nose and causes difficulties in eating and drinking. If a patient

membranes will become excessively dry. Oxygen is only slightly soluble in water, and can be passed through solution with very little loss. Distilled water is used for this purpose. The procedure for moisturizing oxygen differs slightly from one institution to another. In most hospitals, the oxygen is piped into patient rooms, operating rooms, recovery rooms, and

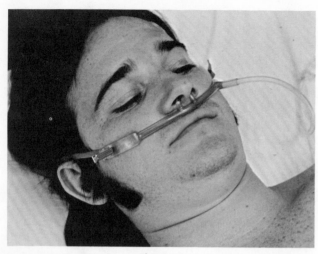

Figure 5-9

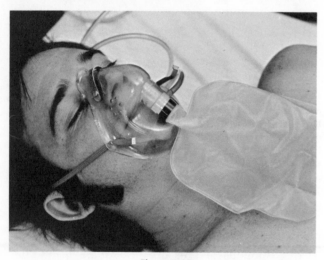

Figure 5-10

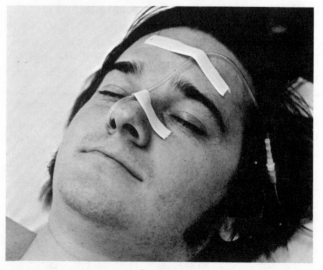

Figure 5-11

Figures 5-9 through 5-11 are from Eunice M. King, Lynn Wieck, and Marilyn Dyer, *Illustrated Manual of Nursing Techniques* (Philadelphia: J. B. Lippincott Company, 1977), pp. 197-98.

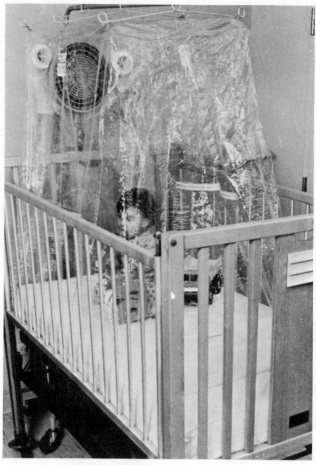

Figure 5-12

is a "mouth breather," however, this may be the only practical method to use (Fig. 5-10).

The nasal catheter is a single french catheter placed in the nostril and inserted into the mouth until it reaches the back of the tongue. It is an efficient but uncomfortable device (Fig. 5-11).

An oxygen tent is a light, portable structure, made of clear plastic, which has a motor-driven unit. The motor circulates the oxygen in the tent. A thermostat inside the tent can be adjusted to suit the patient's comfort. The tent fits over the top of the bed, and the patient's head and chest are inside the tent. This arrangement is used for pediatric patients who would have a difficult time keeping a catheter or mask in place. When the RT must attend a patient who is in an oxygen tent, he may request that the oxygen be turned off for brief periods while he makes his exposures (Fig. 5-12).

Summary

Fever indicates a disturbance in the heat-regulating centers of the body. It can be detected by an elevation in body temperature and can be measured by a clinical thermometer. The body temperature of a normal adult man or woman is 36.7° C (97.6° F) axillary; 37° C (98.6° F) orally; and 38° C (99.6° F) rectally.

The pulse is a reflection of the heartbeat, which sends blood to the arteries and causes the artery to throb. The areas where pulse can be measured best are at the radial artery (radial pulse), the temporal artery (temporal pulse), the carotid artery (carotid pulse), the femoral artery (femoral pulse), the apex of the heart (apical pulse), and the dorsal pedal (pedal pulse). The apical pulse is measured by listening to it through a stethoscope. The average adult male or female has a pulse rate of seventy to eighty beats per minute. The rate changes with age, exercise, or physiological disturbance.

The exchange of oxygen and carbon dioxide between the atmosphere and the blood circulating in the body is accomplished by respiration, which involves the inspiration of air containing oxygen and the expiration of air containing carbon dioxide. The rate of respiration in a normal adult male or female is from sixteen to twenty per minute. Exercise, age, or disease may cause alterations.

Blood pressure is the pressure exerted by the blood on the wall of a blood vessel. It is measured with a sphygmomanometer and a stethoscope. The most practical place to measure blood pressure is at the brachial artery, which is located at the center of the anterior elbow.

To record blood pressure, two readings are noted: the systolic reading is the highest point of pressure reached during a heart contraction, and the diastolic reading is the lowest point reached during a heart contraction. Blood pressure readings, like temperature, pulse, and respiration, are influenced by age, exercise, and disease processes.

Life could not continue without oxygen, yet it cannot be stored in the human body. When a disease process that prevents the body from taking in enough oxygen is present, the needed oxygen must be supplied by artificial means. This may be done in the radiology department in emergency situations, and is frequently done on hospital wards. Oxygen supports combustion, so precautions must be taken when it is in use. No flames or sparks that may produce flame may be used when oxygen therapy is in progress. If the RT must take a radiographic exposure when oxygen is in use, he must make all of his preparations beforehand; in this way the oxygen will be cut off for only a brief moment, if the equipment being used makes this necessary. Oxygen may be administered by nasal cannula, catheter, mask, or tent.

The RT may be responsible for assisting with oxygen administration and for monitoring vital signs in emergency situations in the radiology department, so it is important that he become proficient in these skills.

See Appendix for pre-post test on Chapter 5.

Medical Emergencies in the Radiology Department

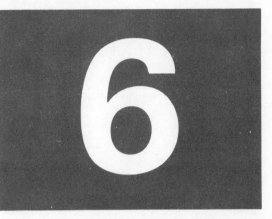

6

Goal of This Chapter
The RT must be able to recognize life-threatening emergencies and be able to initiate the correct medical action.

Objectives
When the RT student has completed this chapter, he will be able to:
1. List four observable symptoms of a patient in a state of shock.
2. List three early symptoms of an anaphylactic reaction.
3. List two symptoms of cardiac failure and describe the action an RT should take if this emergency should occur.
4. List two symptoms of respiratory failure and describe the action an RT should take if this emergency should occur.
5. Describe actions an RT would take if a patient appeared to be having an insulin reaction or was lapsing into a diabetic coma.
6. List the emergency action an RT would take if a patient were having a convulsive seizure or fainting.

Glossary
allergy an oversensitivity to any substance which causes the body to react by producing hives, itching, redness and/or swelling; these reactions may range from mild to severe

anaphylactic shock a serious form of shock due to extreme sensitivity to a drug, a person, or a foreign substance

cardiac pertaining to the heart

cardiac arrest cessation of heart function

cardiogenic originating in the heart

carotid relating to the principal artery of the neck

Many patients come to the radiology department in poor physical condition. This may be due to illness or injury or because of necessary preparation for a particular examination that they will undergo while in the radiology department. When a person is in a weakened physical condition, his physiological reactions may be abnormal. Many of these reactions occur quickly with little or no warning, and they often are life-threatening if not treated immediately.

The abnormal physiological reactions most likely to occur in the radiology department are: fainting, grand mal seizures, insulin reaction, diabetic coma, shock, cardiac failure, and respiratory failure. All are medical emergencies which require immediate action. The RT may be the first member of the health team to observe these reactions; he must be able to recognize their symptoms and to initiate proper action.

Shock
Physical shock is a state in which the heart, respiratory system, and the circulation are disturbed by a major insult to the body. It may be caused by injury, disease, or severe emotional reaction. A patient can lapse into a state of shock very quickly and without warning. For this reason, the RT who is caring for a seriously injured or ill patient must observe closely for any indication of shock. There are several categories into which shock may be subdivided. They will be discussed in the following paragraphs.

Glossary cont.

circumoral around or near the mouth

cyanosis a bluish discoloration of the skin and mucous membranes due to loss of oxygen in the blood

eclampsia convulsion and coma occurring in a pregnant or newly delivered female; rising blood pressure and protein in the urine are warning signals; cause is unknown

edema the presence of abnormally large quantities of fluid in the intercellular (between cells) tissue spaces

epigastric pertaining to the upper-middle region of the abdomen

epilepsy a sudden passing disturbance of brain function that may result in occasional loss of consciousness, abnormal muscle activity, and mental or sensory disturbances

fainting experiencing a temporary loss of consciousness due to loss of blood to the brain

grand mal seizure a sudden loss of consciousness immediately followed by generalized convulsions

histamine an organic compound containing nitrogen sometimes found in body tissues; its three actions are dilatation of capillaries, constriction of bronchial smooth muscle of the lungs, and induction of increased gastric secretion

intracostal on the inner surface of the rib

lethargy a condition of drowsiness or indifference

pallor absence of skin coloration; paleness

parenteral through injection rather than digestive tract

plasma the fluid portion of the blood in which the corpuscles are suspended

prophylactic tending to ward off disease

pulmonary congestion fluid filling the lungs

seizure the sudden attack or recurrence of a disease; an attack of epilepsy

semi-Fowler's a sitting position with the patient's back elevated 45° and the knees elevated 15°

septic produced by or due to decomposition by microorganisms

shock a condition of acute circulatory failure due to derangement of circulatory control or loss of circulating body fluids

systemic affecting the body as a whole

tetanus an infectious disease resulting in trismus (lockjaw), generalized muscle spasm, arching of the back, and seizures

tissue perfusion a liquid poured over or through the tissues of the body

uremia the retention of excessive by-products of protein metabolism in the blood, and the toxic condition produced by it

vital signs signs of life, including body temperature, pulse, respiration, and blood pressure

wheezing making a whistling sound while breathing

HYPOVOLEMIC SHOCK

Hypovolemic shock is caused by an abnormally low volume of circulating fluid (plasma) in the body. It may be due to hemorrhage or burn.

Patient Symptoms and Signs:
- fainting, dizziness, restlessness, anxiety;
- decreased or falling blood pressure;
- weak, thready pulse, and shallow respirations;
- extreme weakness, lethargy, semiconsciousness, coma;
- circumoral pallor and lip cyanosis;
- pale, cool, clammy, cyanotic skin;
- subnormal body temperature;
- possible complaint of excessive thirst and nausea, and vomiting;
- subnormal urinary output.

RT Actions:
- Cardiac failure will follow if this condition is allowed to continue. The RT must act promptly.
- Stop the radiographic examination. Place the patient in the supine position and allow him to rest.
- Note visible body fluid such as bleeding, vomiting, or urination.
- Notify the radiologist immediately.

- Be prepared to assist with administration of oxygen and, if necessary, intravenous fluid.
- Keep patient warm and dry; check blood pressure, pulse, and respiration.
- If there is blood loss from an open wound, apply pressure directly to the wound with a sterile dressing.
- Remain with the patient and provide reassurance.
- Maintain a quiet, nonstressful environment.
- Do not offer the patient food or liquids.
- Any evidence of bleeding should be removed.

SEPTIC SHOCK

Septic shock is caused by a severe systemic infection.

Patient Symptoms and Signs:
- excessive thirst, nausea, vomiting; fainting, dizziness, restlessness, anxiety;
- falling blood pressure, weak and thready pulse, shallow respiration;
- subnormal or elevated temperature;
- lethargy, semiconsciousness, coma;
- cool, or very hot, clammy, cyanotic skin;
- urine output scanty;

- breath sounds diminished;
- possible pulmonary congestion.

RT Actions:

- Stop radiologic examination.
- Place patient in supine position and keep him quiet.
- Do not offer food or any fluid.
- Immediately notify radiologist or physician in charge.
- Take vital signs.
- If skin is very warm to the touch, cover patient with a sheet only.

CARDIOGENIC SHOCK

Cardiogenic shock is caused by a failure of the heart to pump an adequate amount of blood to the vital organs. This causes inadequate tissue perfusion. The onset of cardiogenic shock is sudden and often without warning.

Patient Symptoms and Signs:

- restlessness, anxiety, falling blood pressure;
- weak, rapid pulse and shallow, difficult respirations;
- possible semiconsciousness or coma.

RT Actions:

- Summon assistance and place emergency cart near patient.
- Place patient in semi-Fowler's position or an upright sitting position.
- Take vital signs.
- Be prepared to assist with administration of oxygen.
- Keep patient quiet, and stay with him.

ANAPHYLACTIC SHOCK

Anaphylactic shock is due to a severe allergic reaction. Often the reaction is caused by parenteral administration of a drug that the patient cannot tolerate. It is the type of shock that the RT may see most often in the radiology department because the contrast media used in many procedures may be extremely irritating and therefore produce allergic reactions. When any of these media are being used, the RT must observe the patient carefully for any sign of an allergic reaction.

Patient Symptoms and Signs:

- edema;
- itching at site of injection or around eyes and nose;
- sneezing;
- apprehensiveness.

These symptoms are rapidly followed by:

- edema of face, hands, and other parts;
- wheezing or difficult respirations and cyanosis;
- falling blood pressure, rapid weak pulse, dilated pupils.

Death may follow within a few minutes due to constriction of the smooth muscles by histamine.

RT Actions:

- Keep emergency cart readily available whenever a contrast medium is being administered.
- Before starting any procedure that involves the use of a contrast medium, ask the patient whether he has had any history of allergy. If he has an allergy problem, notify the radiologist before starting the procedure.
- When administering a contrast medium, carefully observe patient for any sign of allergic reaction. If patient complains of itching, or if swelling or redness of skin is noted, immediately stop administering medication and notify the radiologist.
- If patient is in anaphylactic shock, place him in semi-Fowler's or supine position, and be prepared to assist with administration of oxygen and intravenous medication (usually epinephrine).

Diabetic Coma and Insulin Reactions

Diabetes mellitus is a chronic metabolic disease involving a disorder of carbohydrate metabolism that leads to abnormalities of protein and fat metabolism. The underlying cause is a disturbance in the production, action, or utilization of insulin, a hormone secreted by the islands of Langerhans located in the pancreas. Insulin coma and ketoacidosis leading to diabetic coma are the complications the RT must be especially aware of.

A diabetic patient may come to the radiology department after he has taken his daily dose of insulin, but before his body has had sufficient nourishment to utilize the insulin. The result may be an insulin reaction which can range from mild to severe. The onset of symptoms is rapid, and immediate action is necessary to prevent coma.

Patient Symptoms and Signs:

- shaking, nervousness and irritability, dizziness;
- profuse perspiration, cold and clammy skin;
- possible complaint of headache, blurred vision, tremor, numbness of lips or tongue.

RT Actions:

- If patient displays these symptoms and is not a known diabetic, ask the patient if he has a history of diabetes. If insulin reaction is a possibility, quickly obtain sugar or any carbohydrate and insist that the patient eat it. If patient is groggy and unable to swallow normally, place granulated sugar (the kind kept in the lounge for coffee and tea) in his mouth. It will be absorbed by the mucous membranes.

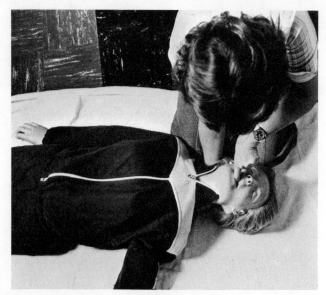

Figure 6-1. Tilt the patient's head back and raise his chin. Examine the patient's mouth for the presence of foreign material which may be obstructing his airway.

- Summon the radiologist immediately. Hypoglycemia must be treated very promptly, because it interferes with oxygen supply to nerve tissue, and this can result in severe brain damage and death.

Ketoacidosis

When a diabetic has insufficient insulin available to metabolize the glucose present, he may lapse into ketoacidosis. In this condition, acid and ketone bodies accumulate in the blood; if it is not corrected quickly, the patient will become comatose and may die. This situation could arise if a diabetic is detained for too long a time in the radiology department and misses an insulin injection.

Patient Symptoms and Signs:
- weakness, drowsiness;
- epigastric pain, nausea and vomiting;
- very dry skin, parched tongue;
- face is flushed, and respirations are deep and rapid.

RT Actions:
- Learn to recognize symptoms—an inexperienced RT may not understand why a diabetic is presenting such symptoms.
- Immediately notify the radiologist.
- Sugar may be given as a prophylactic measure.

Cardiac and Respiratory Failure

Respiratory failure or inadequacy may result from airway obstruction or from physical causes such as pulmonary congestion. A partially obstructed airway may be recognized by noting a patient's difficult breathing or his retracting the intracostal spaces upon inspiration. If a patient is having difficulty breathing, he should be assisted into a sitting or semi-Fowler's position.

There are no symptoms and signs as such. If a patient has lapsed into complete respiratory failure, his pulse beat will continue for a brief period of time. However, the pulse quickly becomes weak and then ceases. The pupils of the eyes dilate and chest movement stops. The observer will be unable to detect air movement through the patient's nose or mouth.

If the RT suspects respiratory failure, he should call for help immediately and then tilt the patient's head back as far as possible by lifting the patient's chin. This maneuver should be omitted if there is a possibility that the patient might have an injury to his neck or cervical spine. If the airway is blocked, this simple movement may re-establish breathing. If it does not, the RT must check the patient's mouth and throat with his finger and remove any foreign material that might be present (Fig. 6-1). If the patient does not resume breathing, then artificial resuscitation must be started at once.

When cardiac failure occurs, the absence of a pulse rate is immediate. The patient loses consciousness immediately and has a deathlike appearance. Breathing is absent and the pupils of the eyes become dilated. The carotid pulse should be checked immediately if cardiac arrest is suspected. If there is no pulse or a questionable pulse, artificial circulation should be started.

Cardiac failure (cardiac arrest) and respiratory failure may occur in the radiology department without any warning when least expected. The RT must take emergency action instantly. The body may survive without oxygen for only two to four minutes, so there is no time to ponder the situation before acting.

The RT must acquaint himself with his department, in order to be able to go directly to the emergency equipment when it is needed. He must know where the emergency drug trays and equipment are kept and how to summon emergency help by the hospital telephone. He should also familiarize himself with the oxygen equipment in his department so that he can assist with its administration.

CARDIOPULMONARY RESUSCITATION (CPR)

All hospital employees, including RTs, are now required to be able to perform basic cardiopulmonary resuscitation (CPR). Many hospitals teach CPR courses on a regular basis to their employees. Others require that the employees take such training in the community. The American Red Cross and the American Heart Association regularly provide these courses for the public. The techniques must be demonstrated by an instructor. Return demonstrations by the student are an important part of this program. The RT must understand that the brief explanation of cardiopulmonary resuscitation that follows does not prepare him to administer cardiopulmonary resuscitation. It is his obligation to his patients to have adequate training in CPR.

If the RT suspects that a patient has had respiratory or cardiac arrest, he must first check the patient's respirations. This is done by observing for chest movement that is present in normal respiration. If no chest movement is seen, put your ear close to the patient's mouth and nose and listen and feel for expiration of air. Next check the carotid pulse and the pupils of the eyes. If there is no sign of breathing, the pulse is absent and the pupils are dilated, call for help and then begin cardiopulmonary resuscitation. Do not wait for help to arrive to begin this. If respirations are absent, but a pulse is felt, begin only pulmonary resuscitation.

Pulmonary resuscitation is begun by hyperextending the patient's neck and pulling the jaw upward. If injury to the neck or cervical spine is suspected, do not do this. In an adult patient squeeze the nostrils together and cover the patient's mouth with your mouth. Inflate the patient's lungs by giving two quick breaths. If this is properly done, the patient's chest will rise as you breathe into his mouth. After this first step, check the carotid pulse once again. If it is present, continue pulmonary resuscitation by breathing into the patient's mouth at the rate of twelve times per minute. If the pulse is absent, cardiac compression is begun.

If the RT is beginning the resuscitation alone, after two breaths, he will begin external cardiac compression. It is effective only if the patient is lying on a firm surface. If the patient is on the radiographic table, kneel on the table beside the patient. If the patient is lying on a soft surface, he should be moved to the floor, or a cardiac board may be placed under the patient's chest.

Place the heel of the hand on the lower third of the sternum, over the heart. The other hand is placed over the first hand. Compress the sternum one and one half to two inches directly downward. Do not compress too low on the sternum or the xiphoid process may cause internal injury. Do not apply pressure on the rib cage itself. Keep your elbows straight and give fifteen sharp compressions, then inflate the patient's lungs two more times. Then give fifteen more compressions. This rhythm must be maintained until help arrives.

If two people are present to administer cardiopulmonary resuscitation, one person will remain

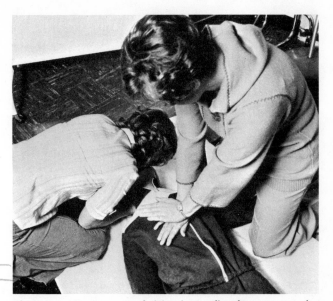

Figure 6-2.   Two persons administering cardiopulmonary resuscitation.

at the head of the patient and inflate the lungs and the other will perform the cardiac compressions. When two people are working together, two lung inflations are given and the carotid pulse is checked. If there is no pulse rate felt, cardiac compression is begun. After every fifth compression, the lungs are inflated one time. There must be sixty cardiac compressions per minute and twelve assisted respirations per minute for an adult victim (Fig. 6-2). The rate of ventilations and the rate and pressure of cardiac compressions will vary in infants and children, depending upon their age and size. The rhythm of this procedure must be regular with never more than five seconds of interruption except for a special procedure such as an intratracheal intubation.

When the emergency team arrives, the RT will allow them to take over and he will remain on the scene to assist with oxygen and drug administration, if this is necessary, or to render service in any way possible.

Fainting and Convulsive Seizures

Fainting and convulsive seizures are medical emergencies which can occur in the radiology department. Both require immediate action to prevent injury to the patient.

FAINTING

Fainting is caused by an insufficiency in the supply of blood to the brain. Hunger, poor ventilation, fatigue, and emotional shock are all causes. For example, patients are frequently instructed not to eat breakfast before coming to the radiology department from their homes or their hospital rooms. Often they are ill, and lack of nourishment may increase the likelihood of fainting. The patient cannot choose the "proper" place in which to faint, so he may fall and injure himself. The RT must be able to recognize and watch for symptoms which indicate that a patient is about to faint.

Patient Symptoms and Signs:
- pallor, dizziness, possibly nausea;
- cold, clammy skin.

RT Actions:
- Have the patient lie down, if possible. Position his head so it is level with or somewhat lower than his body.
- If there is no convenient place where the patient can lie down, do not try to keep him standing, but support and assist him to the floor in a manner that will prevent serious injury. As soon as the patient is in a safe position, summon medical assistance.

CONVULSIVE SEIZURES

Convulsive seizures may be associated with many physical disorders, including uremia, eclampsia, tetanus, infections characterized by high body temperature, poisoning, and increased intracranial pressure due to brain tumors. Epilepsy is the most common cause of convulsive seizures. Children are more susceptible than adults to seizures of all types.

Seizures, like fainting, begin without warning. Though the seizure itself will not cause injury, the patient may be badly injured by falling or because of violent body movement during the seizure.

There are two main types of seizures, known as grand mal and petit mal. A grand mal seizure is one in which the patient's entire body convulses, and he loses consciousness for minutes.

Patient Symptoms and Signs (Grand Mal Seizure):
- may utter a sharp cry as air is rapidly exhaled;
- muscles become rigid and eyes open wide;
- jerky body movements and rapid, irregular respirations;
- may froth, and may have blood-streaked saliva caused by biting his lips or tongue;
- possibly urinary or fecal incontinence;
- usually falls into a deep sleep following the seizure.

For petit mal seizure the attack is so brief an observer may not be aware it has occurred. Though not as frightening to the observer, these seizures may be more difficult to control medically than the grand mal type.

Patient Symptoms and Signs:
- a few jerky movements and momentary loss of consciousness;
- if patient has been addressing someone, may stop speaking, lower his head for a moment, then resume speaking.

RT Actions:
- The most important action is to prevent the patient from injuring himself during a seizure.
- If possible, place the patient in prone position and put a pillow under his head. Do not attempt to insert hard objects such as airways into the patient's mouth. *Do not place your own fingers in the patient's mouth—they may be severely bitten.*
- Stay with the patient. Protect him from hitting his head or limbs against hard objects. Restrain him gently. If he is lying on a radiographic table, hold him. Call for help, but do not leave the patient.

Summary

Medical emergencies occur frequently in the radiology department. The RT may be the first or only person present when they happen, so it is important that he learn to recognize the symptoms of serious problems and know what action to take.

Shock is a common medical emergency. There are many causes for physiological shock. Blood loss, infection, and cardiac failure are among the most common. Anaphylactic shock is caused by allergic reaction and is the one that the RT is most likely to see in the radiology department. Contrast media used for radiologic examinations frequently produce allergic reactions. If early symptoms of this type of reaction are detected, the RT must not wait, but must stop the drug administration immediately. Early symptoms of an anaphylactic reaction are: redness around the eyes, itching, and shortness of breath.

Diabetic coma and insulin reactions are seen in the radiology department because diabetic patients may come for radiologic examinations having taken insulin but not eaten breakfast. This may produce an insulin reaction. Ketoacidosis may occur if a diabetic patient has not had his insulin medication and his body is not able to metabolize the glucose present. Either of these reactions may cause coma and death if the symptoms are not recognized and treated promptly. Sugar in some form must be given and the physician notified.

Cardiac failure and respiratory failure should be differentiated by the RT. Respiratory failure can be recognized by an absence of chest movement and breath sounds and a diminishing pulse rate. Cardiac failure results in immediate absence of pulse rate and loss of consciousness. Both call for immediate action if the patient's life is to be saved.

Fainting and convulsive seizures may develop with little or no warning. The RT should be able to recognize the problem and protect the patient from injuries caused by falls or by hitting the head or extremities against hard surfaces.

The RT must know where the emergency drugs, oxygen, and other supplies are kept in the radiology department. He must also know what action to take if a medical emergency should occur. When the radiologist and other experienced medical personnel have come to the patient's assistance, the RT should stay close by to offer assistance when needed.

See Appendix for pre-post test on Chapter 6.

Care of Patients with Special Problems

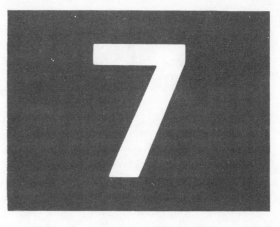

Pediatric patients range in age from one month to fourteen years. Children in this broad age group will require special care, depending upon their age and their ability to understand what is going on. In the RT's initial assessment of each child, he must determine the age of the child and then decide how he will be able to most successfully relate to that child.

The infant will often be accompanied by worried parents. They will be the persons to whom the activities and procedures should be explained. Older children will need a personal explanation. When caring for the pediatric patient in the radiology department, honesty and gentle firmness are important considerations.

A patient who has spinal injuries, a fractured skull, facial injuries, or acute abdominal pain usually is admitted to the emergency room or the radiology department as an extreme emergency case. Such patients need immediate care, but this cannot be started until the diagnostic radiograms are made available to the physician. The RT is taught to make "ideal" exposures, but in emergency cases it may not be possible to do this. He must settle for the best exposures that the situation allows. *The uninformed RT can increase the injury or cause the patient extreme pain and discomfort.* He must therefore exercise great care and understanding when dealing with patients in this category.

The Pediatric Patient

Children of all ages respond to honesty and friendliness. A small child may be very frightened when he enters the radiology department and sees the

Goal of This Chapter

The RT must recognize the need to modify his methods of care when dealing with a young patient or one who has specific injuries.

Objectives

When the student has completed this chapter, he will be able to:
1. List the special considerations necessary when the patient is a child.
2. Demonstrate safe methods of restraining a pediatric patient.
3. List the precautions that must be taken if the patient has a fracture or possible fractures.
4. List precautions to be taken if the patient has symptoms of injury to the spine.
5. List precautions to be taken if the patient has head injuries.
6. List precautions to be taken if the patient has facial injuries.

Glossary

appendicitis   an inflammation of the vermiform appendix

cervical spine   the spinal column at the neck

cholecystitis   inflammation of the gall bladder

ectopic pregnancy   an early pregnancy located away from the normal area; often in the fallopian tube

emesis   vomiting, the act of vomiting

fontanel (fontanelle)   a soft spot such as one of the membrane-covered spaces remaining in the incompletely closed skull of a fetus or infant

fracture   the breaking of a part, especially a bone

Glossary cont.

intravenous pyelogram   a roentgenogram of the kidney and ureter, especially showing the pelvis of the kidney; contrast medium is injected intravenously to demonstrate the area

peripheral nervous system   nerves situated away from the central nervous system

ulcer   a local defect or opening of the surface of an organ or tissue produced by the sloughing of inflammatory dead tissue

---

darkened rooms and the massive equipment. If the RT will spend a few moments acquainting the child with his new environment, he will save himself a great deal of time later. The work will proceed more smoothly and the RT will have a patient who feels secure.

The RT should always explain to the child who is old enough to understand what is going to be done to him. He should explain approximately how long the procedure will last and what will be expected of the patient. The child should be prepared for any discomfort that he may feel. If the child is to receive medication, the method of administration should be explained. Parents who accompany a very young child will be more comfortable if they also are given an explanation. It may be of help to the RT and the parent if parental participation is enlisted. The small child is more responsive to a parent's requests, and will allow the parent to dress him or hold him without feeling the anxiety that might be present if a stranger were to do this. However, department regulations may not permit this type of parental participation.

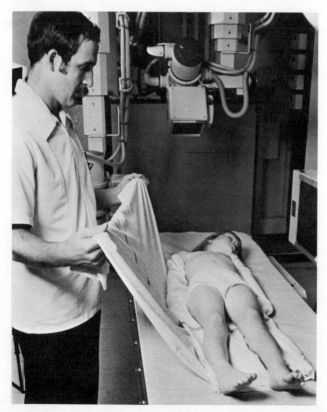

Figure 7-1

Occasionally the very small child or infant will not be able to stay quietly in one place long enough for a successful examination to be completed, and he will have to be restrained. Restraints should be used as a last resort and should be of a type that will not cause injury to the patient. There are several methods of restraining children. Restraints can be fashioned by folding a sheet in a particular manner. There are commercial restraints that are effective for certain procedures. Also, the child may be restrained by being held in position by one or two assistants.

If a child is to be physically restrained by an assistant during a procedure, the RT must instruct the assistant not to be too forceful in his restraining hold. Care should be taken not to pinch or bruise the skin. It is better to use a sheet restraint than to have the assistant place his body over the child because this can be very frightening to the child. To prevent a small child or infant from rolling his head from side to side, the person holding the child should stand at the head of the table and support the child's head between his hands, making sure that he is not pressing on the ears or the fontanels. Any person who holds a child during a radiographic procedure must wear protective lead covering.

Sheet restraints are effective, and can be easily formed in any size or fashion desired. To make a sheet restraint, take a large sheet and fold it lengthwise. Place the top of the sheet at the child's shoulders and the bottom at his feet. Leave the greater portion of the sheet on one side of the child. Bring this longer side back over the arm and under the body and other arm. Next, bring the sheet back over the exposed arm and under the body again. This type of restraint keeps the two arms safely and completely restrained and leaves the abdomen exposed (Fig. 7-1).

Another method of restraint is the mummy style of sheet restraint. This is made by folding a sheet or a blanket into a triangle and placing it on the radiographic table. The distance from the fold to the lower corner of the sheet should be twice the length of the child. Place the child on the sheet with the fold slightly above the shoulders. Loosen or remove the child's clothes. Bring one corner of the sheet over an arm and under the child's body. If both arms are to be restrained, do the same with both sides of the sheet. If the legs are to be restrained, turn the sheet and repeat the procedure for the legs. This restraint can be used

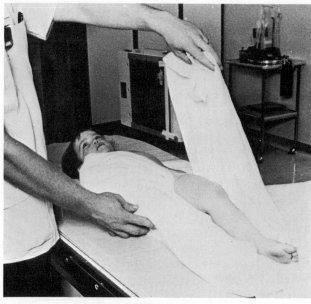

Figure 7-2

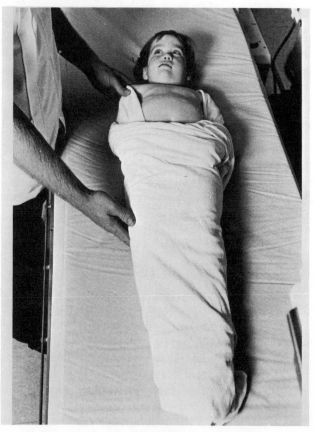

Figure 7-3

to restrain one extremity or all extremities (Figs. 7-2 and 7-3).

There are commercially made restraints that are also recommended. The Pigg-o-stat is a mechanical restraint that is excellent for holding a child safely in an upright position. It is useful for making exposures of the chest or upright abdominal exposures (Fig. 7-4).

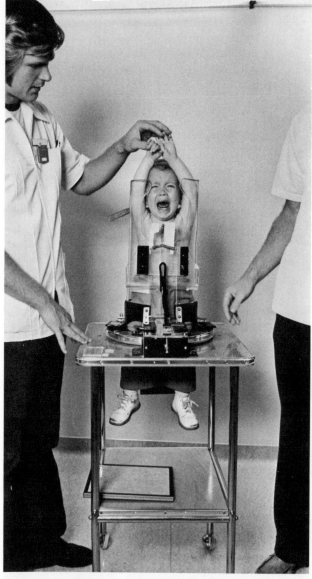

Figure 7-4.   A Pigg-o-stat.   The cassette is inserted into slots directly in front of the patient.

Another restraint is a plastic mold that has straps to hold the extremities. If it is available, this is the best type of restraint for a procedure such as an intravenous pyelogram (Fig. 7-5).

Head Injuries

The RT will be called upon to make radiographic exposures of patients brought to the emergency room with untreated head injuries. These injuries are all potentially serious because of possible involvement of the brain, which is the center of consciousness and is responsible for all of our actions. The brain is made up of soft, moist, spongy tissue which has a rich blood supply. Its protective layer is the skull. With an open injury to the skull, the brain is susceptible to damage because it no longer has a protective casing. If the injury is a closed one, the brain

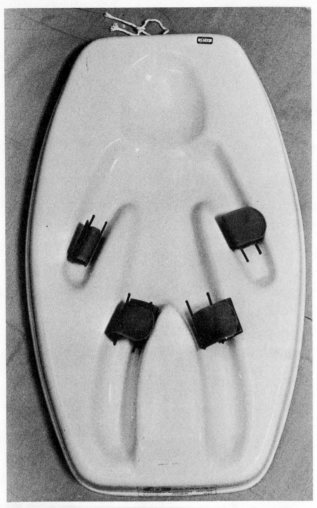

Figure 7-5

obstructed by his tongue. The RT must be aware of this possibility and must check the patient's respiratory rate frequently while working with him.

Spinal Cord Injuries

The spinal cord carries messages from the brain to the peripheral nervous system. It is housed in a canal which extends through the center of the vertebral column. This column is protected by fluid in the canal and by bony structures around the canal. Motor function is dependent upon messages from the brain being transmitted to the spinal nerves on either side of the spinal cord. Injury or severing of the spinal cord causes message transmission to cease. The result is a cessation of motor function and partial or complete cessation of physical function from the level of damage to the cord to all parts below that level. Most spinal cord injuries occur in the cervical or lumbar areas because these are the most mobile parts of the spinal column. The spinal cord loses its protection when there is injury to the protective vertebrae, and such an injury may result in compression or complete severance of the cord. Cord tissue, like brain tissue, has little healing power; injuries to it usually cause permanent damage.

The RT who is called to make radiographic exposures of a patient in whom there is any possibility of spinal injury should not move the patient from the gurney to make these exposures. If the patient must be moved so that good exposures can be made, the physician in charge of the patient must assist with and direct the move.

tissue may swell, but the swelling is limited by the confining skull, and the pressure due to swelling will cause serious brain damage. The brain has little healing power, so any injury to it must be considered potentially permanent and serious. The RT must remember that the patient with a head injury may also have a neck injury.

Often patients with head injuries are unconscious or disoriented, and difficult to manage. In the emergency room, the RT will be caring for these patients after they have been placed on a gurney. *He must never try to change the patient's position in order to make radiographic exposures. The exposures must be made without moving the patient or changing his position in any way.* After the extent of the injury has been determined by the physician, the RT should obtain assistance if it is necessary to move the patient, and should do this under direction of the physician.

The patient with a serious head injury may suffer respiratory arrest. This is a possibility because the gag reflex may be lost or the airway may be

Fractures of the Extremities

Fractures may be classified simply as open or closed fractures. An open fracture indicates a visible wound that extends between the fracture and the skin surface. The broken bone itself often breaks through the soft tissues, making the fracture clearly visible.

A closed fracture may not be obvious to the untrained eye. Often there is swelling around the injured area, pain, and a deformity of the limb. However, all or some of these symptoms may be absent.

If the RT is directed to make radiographic exposures of a fracture or a suspected fracture of an extremity, he must do so without moving the affected limb—to move a patient with either of these types of injuries will cause extreme pain and may compound the damage. Again, if the patient is to be moved, it must be done under direction of and with assistance of the physician in charge of the patient.

Facial Injuries

Injuries to facial bones usually are associated with injury to the soft tissues of the face. Often these injuries are not as serious as they may seem. However, the RT must handle every patient with a facial injury as if the injury were a critical one, because often patients with severe facial injuries have also injured their skull or cervical spine due to the impact of the blow. The unconscious patient may have respiratory failure due to obstruction of the tongue, loose teeth, or bleeding. While the RT is caring for the patient, he must observe the patient's respiratory rate carefully. He must be prepared to take emergency measures if the patient should stop breathing.

All radiographic exposures of patients with facial injuries should be made without moving the patient unless he is ambulatory and communicative. The patient with a serious facial injury should be treated as if he had an injury of the cervical spine or the skull. Any movement should be supervised by the physician in charge of the patient.

Acute Abdominal Distress

There are many reasons for acute abdominal pain. Among them are internal injuries that cause hemorrhage, appendicitis, bleeding ulcers, ectopic pregnancy, cholecystitis, and bowel obstruction.

Whatever the cause of the distress, the symptoms are somewhat similar, and for the RT's purposes, they may be grouped together. The patient is having severe pain and his abdomen often is rigid. Usually he is too ill to be cooperative, so it will be the RT's responsibility to make his radiographic exposures as quickly as possible and with the least possible discomfort to the patient. He may need an assistant to help position and move the patient because the patient will not be able to help. Often several exposures will be ordered and the procedure will take several minutes to complete. If the patient is unable to stand while upright exposures are made, other means of obtaining the radiogram must be considered. Transport the patient by gurney.

The patient with acute abdominal distress may become nauseated and may vomit. An emesis basin and a towel or tissues should be kept nearby. Patients who are hemorrhaging internally often complain of extreme thirst and may request a drink of water. Do not give the patient with acute abdominal pain anything to eat or drink because he may have to be taken to the operating room after a diagnosis is made. It is not safe to anesthetize a patient who has food or fluid in his stomach.

Patients who are hemorrhaging may lapse into hypovolemic shock. The RT should observe the patient with acute abdominal distress for the symptoms of shock. If these symptoms develop, the RT must notify the physician and prepare for emergency treatment of the patient.

Summary

The pediatric patient ranges in age from six weeks to fourteen years. The RT must relate to each age group in an appropriate and specific manner. The infant is usually accompanied by his parent. The RT should ease their anxiety by giving them a brief explanation of the procedure to be performed and how long it will take. Their help in holding the infant should be welcomed and encouraged if it is the policy of the department. The older pediatric patient should be given an honest explanation of his treatment. Forceful restraint of a child should be used only as a last resort. If it is necessary to restrain a child, a restraint made of soft material such as sheeting may be used. If a child is to be restrained by being held, it should be done in a firm, safe manner to prevent injury to the child. An RT should never place his body over a child as a restraint. A sheet restraint or a commercially made one is less traumatic and more effective.

Injuries of the skull, face, spinal cord, and extremities should all be treated as if they were fractures. These injuries are all classified as emergencies, and the RT should make the best radiographic exposure possible without moving the patient. Any movement may cause further injury. If the patient is to be moved, the physician in charge of the patient should assist with and direct the move.

The patient with acute abdominal pain is also classified as an emergency case. These patients are often very ill and are unable to assist the RT. The radiographic exposures should be made as quickly as possible. An assistant should be on hand to help the RT move the patient. The patient may not be able to stand upright while the exposures are made. If this is so, use other methods to obtain desired results. Transport the patient by gurney.

The RT must check the patient with acute abdominal symptoms frequently for signs of hypovolemic shock. The respiratory rate of a patient with face or skull injuries should be checked frequently because he may have respiratory failure. The RT must be able to recognize symptoms of respiratory distress and initiate emergency action if necessary.

Ideal radiographic exposures must be sacrificed in an emergency situation. The best exposure that can be made without moving the patient will have to be acceptable to avoid increasing pain or injury.

See Appendix for pre-post test on Chapter 7.

Administration of Enemas in the Radiology Department

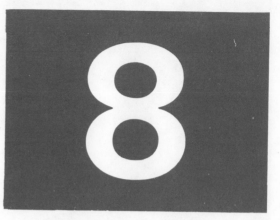

Goal of This Chapter

The RT must have an understanding of the proper technique for administration of enemas and his limitations and responsibilities during this procedure.

Objectives

When the student has completed this chapter, he will be able to:

1. List the precautions that must be taken when administering a cleansing enema and demonstrate the procedure in the laboratory.
2. List the precautions that must be taken when assisting with the administration of a barium enema.
3. Describe special care that must be taken when administering barium enemas to patients with colostomies.

Glossary

carcinoma a malignant growth made up of epithelial cells tending to spread to the surrounding tissues and to give rise to new growths

Chase doll a mannequin which contains all anatomical orifices designed for practice of medical techniques

colostomy the surgical creation of an opening between the colon and the surface of the body

diverticulitis inflammation of a diverticulum (a pouch or sac) created by protrusion of the lining of the mucous membrane through a defect in the muscular coat of a tubular organ

knee-chest position resting upon the knees and chest with forearms supporting the head

lower gastrointestinal tract the lower bowel beginning at the ileocecal junction (the colon)

Cleansing enemas are administered for the purpose of removing feces from the rectum and lower gastrointestinal tract.

Occasionally the RT will be required to administer cleansing enemas in the radiology department if enemas given prior to the patient's arrival there have not been effective. If there is fecal material in the patient's lower bowel, the diagnostic studies will be of very little value. The enema most commonly administered for cleansing purposes is the soap suds enema (SS enema).

Barium enemas are frequently administered in the radiology department to diagnose disorders of the lower gastrointestinal tract. When properly performed, the barium enema is a most effective diagnostic tool. At best, it is very uncomfortable for the patient. If not cautiously performed, it can also be injurious. The RT will be expected to assist frequently with this procedure, so he must know his responsibilities and limitations.

The Cleansing Enema

There are several varieties of cleansing enema. The Fleet enema, the oil retention enema, the tap water enema, and the SS enema are the most common.

The Fleet enema is a commercially prepared enema containing water and Fleet Phospho-Soda. It is packaged in a small plastic container with a pre-lubricated tip. The tip is inserted into the rectum and the liquid is squeezed into the rectum from the plastic

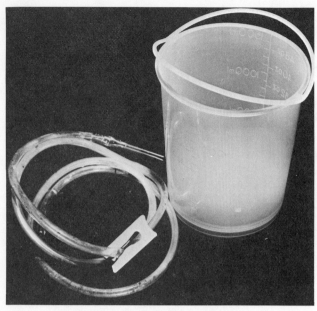

Figure 8-1

bottle. The patient is asked to retain the fluid for several minutes and then to evacuate it. The Fleet enema is quick, easy to use, and effective for relief of constipation and evacuation of the rectum.

The oil retention enema is given for relief of chronic constipation. A small amount of mineral oil or olive oil is instilled into the rectum and the patient is requested to retain the oil for approximately twenty minutes and then to expel it. This type of enema will seldom, if ever, be used by the RT.

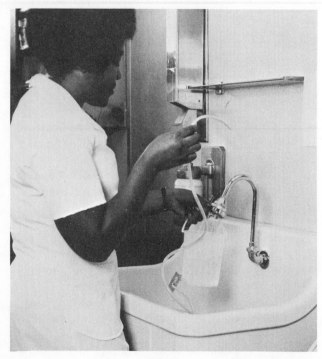

Figure 8-2

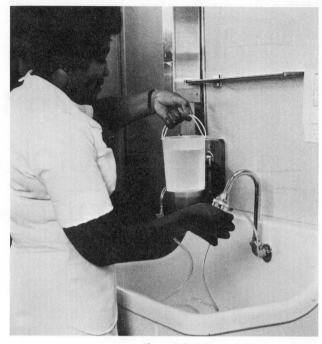

Figure 8-3

Often cleansing enemas for radiographic examinations are administered the night or morning before the examination is to be done. The patient who is not hospitalized may have to do this or have it done at home. The RT must be prepared to give suitable instruction to the outpatient.

The tap water or SS enema is the cleansing enema most frequently used in the radiology department. This procedure is begun by taking an enema set which includes a metal or plastic container that holds 1000 cc. of fluid, a plastic tubing about 4 feet long having a smooth, rounded, perforated tip, and a clamping device (Fig. 8-1). The container is filled with 800 to 1000 cc. of tap water. The temperature of the water is warm, not hot—41-43° C (105 to 110° F) (Fig. 8-2). If soap is to be added, a liquid castile soap is preferred. Add the soap to the water and mix. When the fluid is prepared and the temperature of the water is verified, open the clamp on the tubing and allow the water to run through the tubing into the sink. This allows air in the tubing to be displaced by water and assures that the enema set is working properly. When all air is removed from the tubing, reclamp the tube (Fig. 8-3).

The RT should have ready a terry towel to place under the patient's hips, paper towels, and lubricant for the tip of the tubing. A bed pan should also be placed nearby in case the patient is unable to get to the bathroom to expel the enema. It is most convenient to place all of the items on a tray which can be carried to the patient. Have an area ready on which to place the necessary equipment. If the enema is to be given while the patient is lying on the radiographic table, have a step stool ready for him, so that he can get off the table and get to the lavatory quickly.

When all of the equipment is prepared, approach the patient and explain what is to be done. Arrange for privacy. Keep the patient covered except for body parts that must be visible. Ask him to turn onto his left side (Sims's position) (Fig. 8-4). Lift the buttock and expose the anus, being certain that the exposure is adequate. Lubricate the tip of the tube and insert it through the anal sphincter (usually 2 to 3 inches), at an angle pointing toward the umbilicus (Fig. 8-5). Instruct the patient to take several deep breaths through his mouth while the tip is being inserted.

When the tip is properly inserted, hold it in place with one hand. With the other hand, unclamp the tube and raise the container about 18 to 24 inches above the anus. A standard such as the type used in hanging bottles of intravenous fluid may be used to hold the enema set if it can be adjusted to the correct height. Allow the water to flow in slowly. Instruct the patient to tell you if he has abdominal cramping. If he does, pinch the tube closed until the cramping has passed. Then allow the fluid to continue flowing. For cleansing of the transverse and ascending colon, the patient may be asked to turn onto his right side after the fluid has been instilled. The knee-chest position may be ordered by the patient's physician because it helps promote thorough cleansing of the bowel.

The quantity of fluid that a patient can retain varies, but at least 500 cc. should be administered before the enema is stopped. Instruct the patient to tell you when he has taken as much as he can hold. Clamp the tube before the water has reached the bottom of the container so that air will not enter the rectum. Remove the tube slowly from the rectum. Place the tip of the tube into the container, and set the container aside. Assist the patient to a supine position, then help him walk to the lavatory. If he is not able to go to the lavatory, place him on a bedpan.

While the patient is expelling the enema, the RT can clean the equipment or dispose of it and wash his hands. Instruct the patient not to flush the commode until the expelled material has been observed. The quantity, color, and consistency of the fecal material should be noted.

Barium Enema

Barium enemas are used in diagnosis of pathology of the lower gastrointestinal tract. The patient must begin preparation for this procedure twenty-four hours before it is to be done. His diet should be restricted the previous day to low-residue

liquids. Cathartics are usually prescribed the afternoon before the examination. These are followed by enemas "until clear." This means that enemas are administered either by the patient himself if he is an outpatient, or by a nurse if he is a hospital patient. They are given and expelled until there is no further fecal material. If the fecal matter is not properly cleansed from the large bowel, the examination is of no value and the patient will either be given another cleansing enema in the department or will be required to return on another day. For patients whose physical

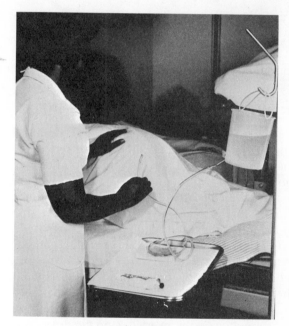

Figure 8-4

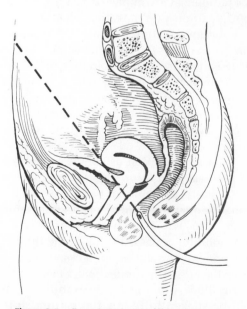

Figure 8-5.   From LuVerne Wolff Lewis, *Fundamental Skills in Patient Care* (Philadelphia: J. B. Lippincott Company, 1976), p. 283.

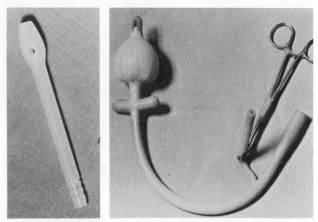

Figure 8-6   Figure 8-7

condition does not permit this rigorous preparation, less than "ideal" preparation may be accepted.

A much larger catheter is required than is used for a cleansing enema. The catheter may have a plain tip or one with an inflatable balloon attached. The balloon is inflated after the tip is inserted, to hold the catheter in place and prevent involuntary expulsion of barium (Figs. 8-6 and 8-7). The RT will usually insert the rectal catheter. The procedure is much the same as for the cleansing enema. The patient is placed in the Sims's position, and the anus is exposed. The tip of the catheter or tube is lubricated generously. Instruct the patient to take short panting breaths while the catheter is being inserted. Insert the tip of the catheter about 3 inches or until it has passed the anal sphincter. Do not use force to insert this catheter. If it cannot be easily inserted, stop the procedure and ask the radiologist to complete it. Return the patient to a supine position after the catheter has been inserted.

Often a retention catheter is used for a barium enema. This type of catheter has a balloon that is inflated after insertion to hold the catheter in place. The balloon may be inflated with a hand inflation pump or a syringe. The RT must be certain that the balloon is inserted beyond the rectal sphincter before inflation. Then inflate initially with no more than 50 cc. of air.

Barium solution usually is available in pre-pared pre-packaged form. The RT should have ready for use a plastic container of barium which has been shaken. The quantity needed for an adult examination generally is 1500 cc., though it may vary (Fig. 8-8). The barium solution is passed through the tubing in the same manner as a solution for a cleansing enema, to displace the air in the tubing before inserting the tip. As described, premixed preparations of barium should be shaken to re-mix the barium so that the suspension is uniform and should be administered at room temperature.

The bag containing barium is hung from a metal standard; a clamp on the tubing opens and closes the tubing easily. The bag should be placed about 30 inches above the table. The RT must not begin instillation of the barium until the radiologist is present in the room to direct the procedure (Fig. 8-9).

Every effort must be made by the RT to keep the patient as comfortable as possible during this examination. The patient should be told that he will be required to move about on the table for various exposures and that the radiologist will be calling instructions to the RT. The patient may mistakenly think that these instructions are meant for him. Each instruction consists of a single word—"open," "close," "off," "on"—and does not refer to the patient directly. The patient should also be informed of the approximate quantity of barium that he will be expected to hold and that a series of radiograms will be needed.

Air is sometimes placed into the bowel during this examination. If this is to be done, it must be done by the radiologist. Barium is instilled first and

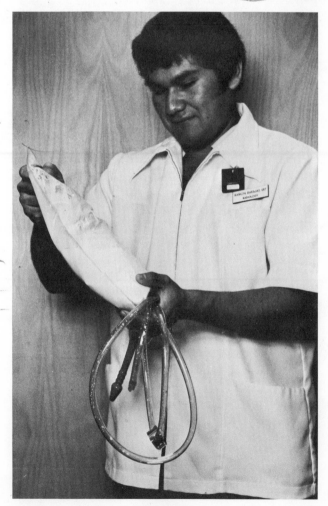

Figure 8-8

the patient is then allowed to evacuate some of the barium. A rectal catheter with an air-insufflating mechanism attached is then inserted and air is injected as a contrast medium. The patient will be extremely uncomfortable during this examination. The RT should remain close to the patient in order to help him move about and assist him in getting to the bathroom when the examination is completed.

When removing a rectal catheter that has a balloon attached, the RT must be certain that the balloon is deflated before removing the catheter. The barium is sometimes removed by gravity flow before the catheter tip is removed, and the air is permitted to escape from the balloon. The RT then gently pulls on the catheter. If there is any resistance, the procedure should be stopped and the radiologist summoned.

The Patient with a Colostomy

A colostomy is a surgical procedure done to treat obstruction of the large bowel. The most common reasons for a colostomy are carcinoma of the colon and severe diverticulitis. The surgical proce-

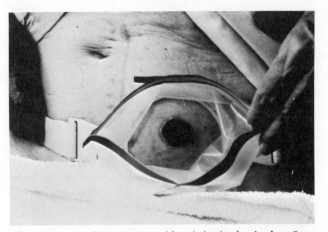

Figure 8-10. A colostomy stoma with an irrigation bag in place. From LuVerne Wolff Lewis, *Fundamental Skills in Patient Care* (Philadelphia: J. B. Lippincott Company, 1976), p. 287.

dure most frequently done is to bring a loop of transverse colon into the surgical wound and partially close the incision, thus creating the colostomy. The colostomy may be a temporary one done to rest diseased bowel, or a permanent one done when diseased bowel must be removed.

A patient who has a colostomy may require barium enemas for further diagnosis. The RT should be aware that the patient will be very concerned and sensitive about his condition and must be treated in a friendly, matter-of-fact manner. It is suggested that the RT who has never seen a colostomy should simply observe the procedure being performed until he can deal with these patients easily.

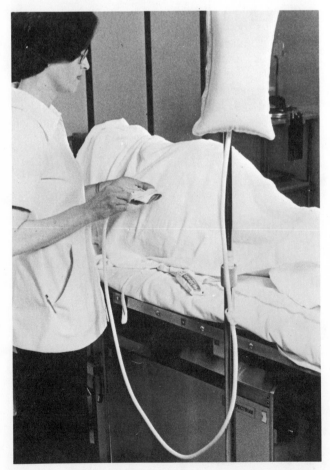

Figure 8-9. The catheter tip should be heavily lubricated with a water-soluble lubricant before it is inserted for a barium enema.

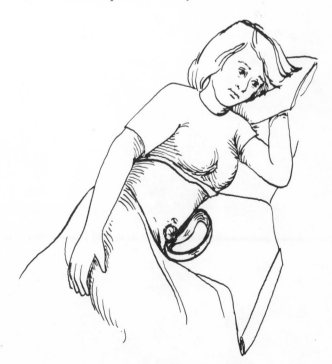

Figure 8-11. Colostomy draining.

The patient will usually have a dressing or a drainage bag in place over the area of his stoma. The dressing must be removed, then may be discarded after being wrapped in newspaper or paper towels. A drainage bag should be removed and put aside safely to be re-used. The patient can usually direct the RT in its care. The bag must be kept clean and dry (Fig. 8-10).

A small catheter with an inflatable balloon is inserted into the colostomy by the radiologist or an experienced technologist. A Foley catheter is most often chosen for this purpose. Disposable gloves may be worn when doing this procedure. The patient is placed in the supine position. The catheter is well lubricated and may be inserted 4 to 5 inches. The radiologist will inflate the balloon on the catheter. Less barium is needed for the patient with a colostomy, 500 cc. usually being the maximum quantity.

Once the catheter has been inserted, the procedure is the same as with all other patients. Barium must not be instilled until the radiologist is present to supervise.

When the procedure is completed, barium may be drained by gravity flow. The patient may then be taken to the lavatory with the catheter still in place, if his physical condition permits. This prevents the barium solution from running out prematurely. The catheter is deflated and gently removed from the colostomy. The patient may expel the barium into a large kidney basin. A second basin should be available for use after the first one is filled.

The patient who is unable to go to the lavatory should be placed on his side and a large kidney basin should be held close to his body just under the colostomy while the barium is being expelled. Have a second basin close by to be used when necessary (Fig. 8-11).

After the barium has been evacuated, a clean dressing should be placed over the colostomy. If the patient attends to his own colostomy, any articles he needs should be made available to him.

Summary

Cleansing enemas are used in the radiology department to complete preparation for administration of barium enemas. There are several types of cleansing enemas; the ones most frequently used in the radiology department are the tap water and SS enemas. The RT must familiarize himself with the steps to be followed in administering a cleansing enema.

The barium enema is an important diagnostic procedure and is performed frequently. A rectal catheter with an inflatable balloon is used to prevent spontaneous evacuation of the barium solution. The RT must be aware of the extreme discomfort that results from this procedure and make the patient as comfortable and relaxed as possible. The inflatable balloon on the catheter and the air insufflated into the bowel as a contrast medium must be instilled by the radiologist.

The patient with a colostomy may also need a barium enema for diagnosis. A smaller catheter is most commonly used for these patients. It has an inflatable balloon to prevent expulsion of barium and is smaller than rectal catheters used for this procedure. Much less barium is used for the colostomy patient. The radiologist must always supervise the procedure.

See Appendix for pre-post test on Chapter 8.

Care of the Patient with a Gastric Tube

9

Goal of This Chapter

The RT student must know how to assist with insertion and care of gastric tubes.

Objectives

When the student has completed this chapter, he will be able to:

1. Prepare a patient for passage of a gastric tube.
2. Transfer a patient with a gastric tube in place from the hospital ward to the radiology department.
3. Care for a patient in the radiology department who is having continuous gastric suction.

Glossary

gastric pertaining to, affecting, or originating in the stomach

gavage forced feeding, especially through a tube passed into the stomach

Gomco suction an electrically operated machine that is attached to a gastric tube to provide continuous drainage from the stomach

lumen the cavity of a tubular organ or the bore of a tube

nasogastric tube a tube that goes from the nose through the esophagus into the stomach

peristalsis the wormlike movements by which the digestive tract or other tubular organs with longitudinal and circular muscle fibers propel their contents

Gastric suction is used both pre- and post-operatively to keep the stomach free of all gastric contents and gas until the stomach and upper gastrointestinal tract heal. Before gastric suction can be used, a gastric tube must be passed into the stomach and occasionally on into the duodenum or small intestine. After the tube is passed, it is attached to an electrical suction apparatus. This suction is maintained either continuously or intermittently as the patient's needs require.

The Gomco thermatic pump is the most common portable suction device used in hospitals today. Many hospitals have suction piped into patient rooms and other rooms or departments where it might be required.

In the radiology department, diagnostic studies are done that involve passage of gastric tubes prior to the examination. The RT will not be called upon to pass these tubes, but he will be asked to prepare the patient. He must understand what type of tube to obtain and what accessory articles will be needed for the procedure.

Transferring the Patient with a Gastric Tube

The RT who is to transfer a patient with a gastric tube should make certain of the doctor's orders before making the transfer. If it is permissible to discontinue the suction, he must know for how long a time it can be stopped. If it is for only a short time, he

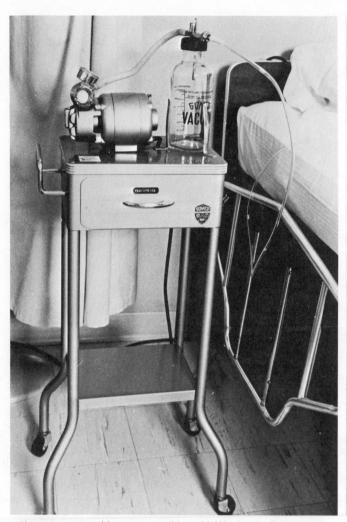

Figure 9-1. Portable suction machine which is electrically operated. The pressure control valve and the pressure indicator are located above the motor. The drainage runs into the vacuum bottle on the right. The tubing at right, is connected to the gastric tube.

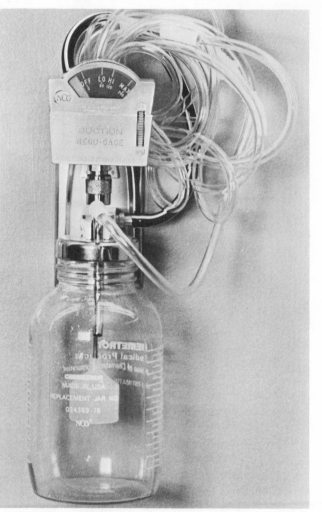

Figure 9-2. Suction equipment is often used in radiology departments, and may be piped to the department from a central area in the hospital. It is activated by turning the valve at the top, right, below the pressure gauge. The suction pressure is regulated by adjusting the valve, center, above the vacuum collecting bottle.

must be certain that suction can be re-established in the radiology department. This can be accomplished by taking the patient's suction machine with the patient or by using the suction in the department if it is available. The RT must also know the amount of suction pressure that is required so that he can adjust the machine properly. The wrong amount of suction pressure may harm the patient (Figs. 9-1 and 9-2).

Clamping a nasogastric tube is a simple procedure, but medical aseptic technique must be followed. The RT may obtain a simple clamping device from the nurse's station on the ward. A package of sterile gauze pads and two rubber bands will also be needed. Disconnect the gastric tube from the adapter that attaches it to the suction machine. Clamp the tube (Fig. 9-3). Allow the gastric contents in the tubing to drain into the drainage bottle. Clamp the gastric tube with a clamp and place one gauze pad over the end of the tubing. Secure it with a rubber band. Place the

second gauze pad over the adapter to keep it clean, in such fashion that it does not fall to the floor (Fig. 9-4). Be certain that the tube is securely taped to the patient's face before moving him. Then proceed with the transfer by wheelchair or gurney as required.

If suction is to be resumed when the patient reaches the radiology department, reconnect the tubing to the suction immediately. Set the suction pressure at the required setting. Unclamp the tubing and turn on the machine. This procedure is repeated when transferring the patient back to his room.

Assisting with Passage of Gastric Tubes

The gastric tubes that are most commonly seen in the radiology department are the Levin tube and the Cantor tube. There are many other gastric tubes, but their purposes and methods of insertion

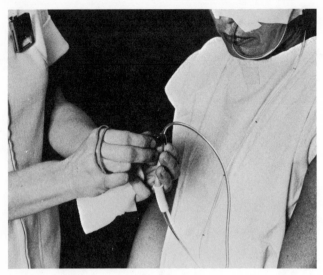

Figure 9-3

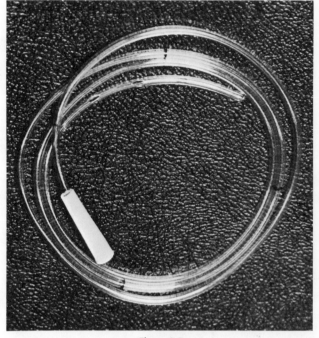

Figure 9-5

are similar. A contrast medium may be instilled into the gastrointestinal tract by means of these tubes to trace their position in the gastrointestinal tract.

The Levin tube is a long plastic or rubber tube which is inserted through the nose or mouth into the stomach. It is used for gavage and to drain off gastric fluids to keep the stomach decompressed (Fig. 9-5).

When diagnosis of gastrointestinal disease necessitates passage of a gastric tube, the RT must prepare the patient and the materials needed.

He must first ascertain what type of tube is needed. If the tube is a rubber tube, it should be placed in a basin of ice. This makes the rubber more rigid and allows for easier passage. Plastic tubes usually are rigid and do not need to be chilled.

The other items needed are: an emesis basin, a glass of water, tissues, adhesive tape, and water-soluble lubricant. A 20 or 50 cc. aspirating syringe will also be needed.

This procedure is uncomfortable and frightening for the patient. The RT should explain what is going to be done and for what reason. The patient should be assured that if he keeps swallowing and breathing deeply the procedure will go smoothly. If swallowing is difficult for the patient, he can be given ice chips or sips of water to aid him in swallowing.

The patient should be placed in Fowler's position if it is possible. If not, the supine position will be satisfactory. Give the patient an emesis basin to hold. If he gags he may use it. If the patient cannot hold the emesis basin, keep it close by. Measure the distance from the nose to the approximate area of the stomach externally before starting the procedure (Fig. 9-6). Levin tubes have black markings at the distal end to help indicate how far the tube has been inserted. The first mark or ring usually indicates that the tube is in the stomach; the second, the pylorus; and the third, the duodenum.

When the radiologist or nurse is ready to insert the gastric tube, the RT may moisten it in water

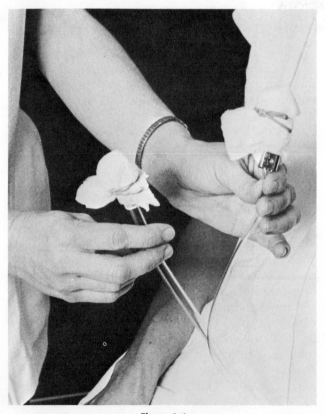

Figure 9-4

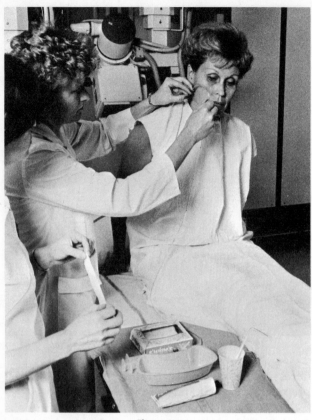

Figure 9-6

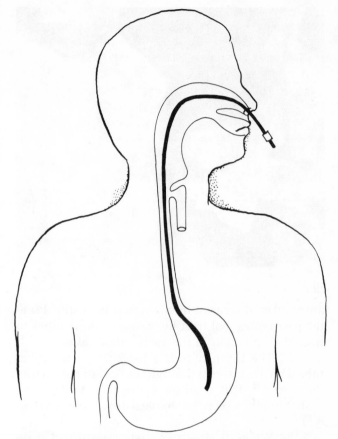

Figure 9-7. Diagram to illustrate position of the Levin tube in the stomach.

and hand it to him. A nostril is the most desirable site of insertion, but if the patient has a deviated nasal septum this may not be the best point of insertion. The mouth, over the tongue, is the second choice. The tube should go down easily and without force.

After insertion of the tube has begun, give the patient sips of water to aid in swallowing. Continually urge the patient to swallow and reassure him while the procedure is in progress.

When the physician or nurse believes that the tube is in the stomach, he can place the tip of the tube on the aspirating syringe and draw back. He should draw up gastric juices into the syringe. If he does not, the tube may be in the trachea. To determine this, place the free end of the tube in a glass of water. If it bubbles, it is in the trachea and should be removed at once. If the patient becomes cyanotic during the procedure, it is also an indication that the tube is in the trachea and must be removed and re-inserted.

When it is certain that the tube has reached the stomach, reassure the patient that the procedure is completed. Then tape the tube, across the bridge of the nose or on the patient's cheek. If the tube is to remain in place for a long time, the most comfortable way of arranging the tube for the patient should be determined. If the tube is to be connected to a suction device, it can be done at this time (Fig. 9-7).

Gastric and Intestinal Decompression Tubes

These tubes are longer than the Levin tube, have an inflatable bag at the end, and may be radiopaque. They are meant to be passed into the duodenum and the small intestine, to relieve distention in the lower gastrointestinal tract, and for diagnostic purposes.

The Cantor tube is an intestinal decompression tube. Because it is frequently used in radiologic procedures, it is a useful example. Before the Cantor tube is inserted, 5 to 9 cc. of mercury is injected into the center of the bag or balloon via a sterile syringe of proper size with a sterile 21-gauge needle. All air should be aspirated from the bag.

The bag is lubricated with a water soluble lubricant and folded lengthwise for insertion through the nose or mouth. To aid insertion, a lubricated cotton-tipped applicator or a bayonet forceps may be used. While still encased in its plastic wrapper, the tube may be placed in hot water to make it more flexible for insertion.

Gastric and intestinal decompression tubes are often inserted before the patient arrives in the radiology department. If the RT does aid in inserting the tube, he must remember not to tape the tube to the patient's face, because this would prevent the movement required to pass the tube into the lower gastrointestinal tract by means of peristalsis. The physician, rather than a nurse, will often insert this type of tube.

On occasion, mercury from the balloon may escape into the gastrointestinal tract. This is of no great significance because metallic mercury is nontoxic and will pass normally (Fig. 9-8).

Removal of Gastric Tubes

The removal of a Levin tube is a simple procedure and can be accomplished easily. The RT may do this with orders from the radiologist. An emesis basin, tissues and several paper towels to receive the tube will be needed.

Explain to the patient what is about to be done. Wash your hands. Remove the tape if there is any holding the tube in place, then slowly withdraw the tube until all of it has been removed. If there is any resistance, call the radiologist to assist. Discard the tube wrapped in paper toweling. Wash your hands and make the patient comfortable.

The Cantor tube and other tubes of this type must be removed very slowly. Rapid removal may cause the patient to gag or vomit, or may cause injury. The tube is withdrawn at intervals. If there is resistance, time must be allowed for it to be released by peristalsis. These tubes will be removed by a nurse or the radiologist.

Care of the Gastric Tube

Patients with gastric tubes in place are very uncomfortable. They should be reassured frequently and not left alone until they feel secure.

The RT must take care to tape the Levin tube securely so that it is not accidentally withdrawn. It should never be necessary to repeat passage of a gastric tube because of careless handling. There should be no pressure pulling the tube. Patients with gastric tubes in place are not to eat or drink anything unless it is specifically ordered.

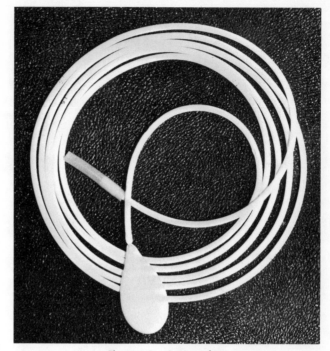

Figure 9-8.   Cantor tube.

Summary

Before transferring a patient with a gastric tube and continuous gastric suction, the RT must learn whether it is permissible to discontinue the suction and for how long a period of time. The patient should be moved carefully. If the suction is continuous it must be re-started, as soon as the patient reaches the radiology department, at the same pressure as was used in his room.

The gastric tubes most often used in the radiology department are the Levin tube and the Cantor tube. The Levin tube enters the stomach, the Cantor, the small intestine. The RT must learn to assist with their passage and care.

Levin tubes may be removed by the RT. They should be removed slowly and without force. Cantor tubes should be removed by a nurse or the radiologist. They are removed slowly and at intervals.

See Appendix for pre-post test on Chapter 9.

Aseptic Technique for the Radiologic Technologist

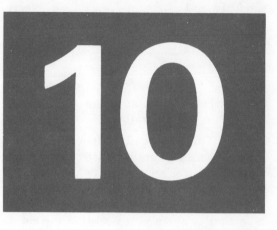

Goal of This Chapter

The RT student will understand the reasons for surgical asepsis and be able to create and maintain a sterile field when it is called for in his department or in the operating room.

Objectives

When the student has completed this chapter, he will be able to:

1. Define surgical asepsis.
2. List the most common means of transmitting microorganisms in the operating room.
3. List the methods of sterilization and the rules for surgical asepsis.
4. Demonstrate, in the laboratory, the correct method of opening a sterile pack to prevent contamination.
5. Demonstrate, in the laboratory, the correct method of placing a sterile object on a sterile field.
6. Demonstrate, in the laboratory, the correct method of putting on a sterile gown and gloves.

Glossary

asepsis   the prevention of contact with microorganisms

disinfect   freeing from infection

don   to put on an article of clothing

fan fold   to fold an article (usually a sheet) upon itself so as to pleat it

fomite   an article (such as a glass or an instrument) which harbors microorganisms

sterile field   an area protected from microorganisms usually by a sterile sheet or covering onto which sterile objects may be placed

Surgical asepsis must be differentiated from medical asepsis. Medical asepsis was discussed in Chapter 2, where it was defined as any practice which helps reduce the number and spread of microorganisms. Surgical asepsis refers to the complete removal of all microorganisms and their spores from the surface of any article or object where they may exist. This practice begins with cleaning the object in a medically aseptic way. It is followed by a sterilization procedure utilizing either heat or chemical action to accomplish the total removal of microorganisms and spores.

Any medical procedure that involves penetration of the skin requires the use of surgical aseptic technique. This includes major and minor surgical procedures, parenteral administration of medications, catheterization of the urinary bladder, and dressing changes.

Many procedures performed in radiology involve penetration of the patient's skin; therefore, they must be done using surgical aseptic technique. Frequently, the RT is called to the operating room for radiographic examinations while a major surgical procedure is in progress. He must be able to do his work in the operating room without contaminating the surgical field.

The RT frequently participates in procedures that call for his knowledge of surgical asepsis. If he is not skilled in its use, he may be responsible for contaminating a surgical field. This causes loss of time while the field is made sterile again. If the contamination is not recognized, microorganisms may be introduced into a surgical wound causing infection. This is a threat to the patient's life or physical well-being.

Glossary cont.

surgical asepsis   practices which keep objects and articles free from all microorganisms and spores

vector   a carrier, especially an animal or insect which transfers an infective agent from one host to another

How Microorganisms Are Spread in the Operating Room

The RT student may recall that microorganisms are spread by direct or indirect contact. Direct transmission occurs when the exposed person is touched by the carrier of the microorganism. The contact is indirect if the microorganism is transferred by means of a fomite, a vector, or the air.

A fomite is any article to which microorganisms cling. These can be dishes, instruments, soiled dressings, and so on. A vector is an animal or an insect that carries microorganisms to a person. Microorganisms can also be blown from place to place by drafts from open doors or by air-conditioning units.

The patient in the radiology department or operating room is easy prey to microorganisms. He is usually in a weakened physical state, and his protective coat—his skin—is being penetrated by needles, catheters, or surgical instruments. Extreme care must be taken in these situations to keep all equipment sterile. All persons working in the operating room change from their outer clothing into special operating room garments called "scrub suits" before entering the operating suite. Hands and forearms are scrubbed for ten minutes in a specified manner with a brush and surgical soap before the person enters the operating room area. Hair must be covered with a surgical cap at all times.

A clean surgical mask is worn over the mouth and nose when an operation or other sterile procedure is going on. Doors are kept closed and air vents are situated so that air does not flow in the direction of the sterile instruments or the operating table. The RT who must use radiographic equipment in the operating room must clean it with an antiseptic solution before taking it into the area. Many hospitals have radiographic equipment that is never removed from the operating suite and is cleaned routinely after every use.

Persons who are actually involved in performing surgical procedures must scrub for ten minutes. When this is completed, they dry their hands with a sterile towel and then dress in a sterile gown and put on sterile gloves. The person dressed in sterile attire and participating in a sterile procedure is sometimes called the "sterile person." One might also say that the person is "scrubbed." After a person is "sterile" or "scrubbed," he may not touch anything that is not sterile. If he does, he is considered contaminated and must change whatever has been contaminated so that it is sterile once again.

The individual who assists the "sterile" person or persons is called the "circulating nurse" or "circulating attendant." This person wears only a scrub suit and a cap and mask and obtains equipment necessary for the procedure and places it on the sterile field in a manner that maintains its sterility. A sterile field is the area that has been prepared for sterile equipment and instruments. It is touched only by the sterile person or persons.

Any break in sterile technique increases the patient's chances of becoming infected. Persons who are involved in a sterile procedure must be constantly aware of which areas and objects are sterile. If a sterile object is touched by an unsterile object, it must be replaced by one that is sterile. A contaminated area must be made sterile again. Proper sterilization techniques must be learned and followed. Proper methods of opening sterile packs and donning sterile gown and gloves must also be learned.

Use of contaminated instruments or gloves, allowing a sterile field to become wet or damp, and allowing microorganisms to be blown onto a surgical site are the most common methods of contamination. With care, they can be prevented.

Methods of Sterilization

There are several methods of sterilization:
1. Dry heat. This can be used when moist heat is inadvisable. It is a slow and uneven method. The length of time it takes to sterilize with dry heat varies from one to six hours. This method is rarely followed.
2. Boiling. This is a moist heat method. It was commonly used in the past and it is still an acceptable means of disinfection. However, infectious hepatitis organisms are resistant to this method, which makes it unacceptable for sterilization in the hospital.
3. Steam under pressure. This has become the most effective and convenient means of sterilization for items that can withstand high temperatures. It is done in an autoclave. The chief advantage of this

method is that higher temperatures can be reached with moist heat. The increased pressure in itself has no effect on the sterilization process. The steam settles on the cold surfaces of the objects in an autoclave and coagulates the protein on them, thus destroying all microorganisms. The steam must reach every surface to be effective. Indicators are placed in the center and outside of each pack to be sterilized. When the indicator changes color, it is proof of the sterilization of the pack contents. There are many variations in these indicators. Most of them change from a light to a dark color. The RT must learn which indicator his department uses and how to read it.

4. Chemicals. This is not a satisfactory method of sterilization. At best, chemicals may disinfect items that cannot be autoclaved. There are limitations with all disinfectants, the chief one being that there is no means of ensuring sterility. If a chemical disinfectant must be used, the directions for its use must be carefully followed, such as the length of time the object must be immersed in the solution, the correct temperature, and the strength of the solution.

5. Gas. This is the method of choice for sterilizing items that cannot withstand high temperatures. A mixture of freon and ethylene oxide is used. An autoclave is heated to 57.3°C (135°F) with a humidity of 50 percent. This humidity is lower than is achieved with steam under pressure. The gas mixture kills both microorganisms and their spores. Gas sterilization may be used for most items; however, because of the length of time required to aerate porous items to remove gas residue, it is reserved for use on glass syringes, lens instruments, rubber catheters, radios and telephones used in isolation rooms, and electrical equipment.

Rules for Surgical Asepsis

When the RT participates in sterile procedures, he must know which areas and objects are sterile and which are not. Sterile objects and persons must be kept separate from those that are unsterile. When anything that must be sterile becomes contaminated, the contamination must be remedied immediately.

Many procedures done in the radiology department are sterile procedures. Some of these are angiography, arteriography, myelography, and arthrography. All injections are also sterile procedures. Most of the sterile equipment for special radiographic procedures comes pre-packaged in airtight, water-

proof containers. Items prepared in the central supply department of the hospital are wrapped in double cloth wrappers, taped with indicator tape, and then sterilized. When paper drapes are used, a single thickness is acceptable. All sterile items should be kept stored in the same place. Unsterile objects must be stored separately from sterile ones.

Furniture and people cannot be "sterilized" in the sense of the word as used in this book. When table tops are to be used as areas for creating a sterile field, they must be clean and a sterile drape must be placed over them. Personnel must be clothed in sterile gowns and gloves to be considered sterile.

If a sterile instrument or a sterile area is touched by an unsterile object or person, it is contaminated by microorganisms. A contaminated area on a sterile field must be covered by a sterile towel or drape of double thickness. If a sterile person's gown or gloves become contaminated, these must be changed. Once a sterile field has been prepared, it should not be left unattended, because it may become contaminated accidentally without being observed.

When there is any question about the sterility of an object, it is to be considered unsterile and must be replaced. An unsterile person must not reach across a sterile field. A sterile field ends at the level of the table top or at the waist of a person's sterile gown. Anything that drops below the table top or a sterile person's waistline is no longer sterile.

The only part of a gown considered sterile is the area from waist to shoulder in front, including the sleeves. No part of the back of the gown is sterile. The edges of sterile wrappers are not considered sterile and must not touch a sterile object. Sterile persons must stay within the sterile area. If a sterile person must pass another person, each must pass the other back to back. The sterile person faces the sterile field. The sterile person keeps his sterile gloved hands above his waist and in front of his chest. He touches only sterile objects.

Any sterile material or packs that become dampened or wet are not considered sterile. Any objects wet with bactericides that are to be placed on a sterile field must be placed on a folded sterile towel to absorb the moisture. A wet area on a sterile field must be covered with several thicknesses of dry sterile towels or drapes.

All areas that are used for sterile procedures should be well cleaned with germicidal solution after each procedure. Floors should be cleaned with a germicide after each procedure. Mops should be of the disposable variety and should be used only once.

Air-conditioning units must be kept clean, and the filters should be changed frequently because they may blow bacteria onto a sterile field.

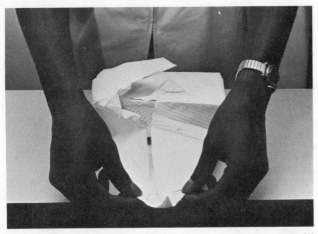

Figure 10-1. Figures 10-1 through 10-3 are from LuVerne Wolff Lewis, *Fundamental Skills in Patient Care* (Philadelphia: J. B. Lippincott Company, 1976), pp. 295-96.

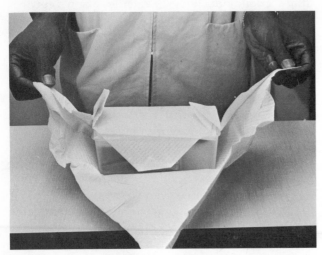

Figure 10-2

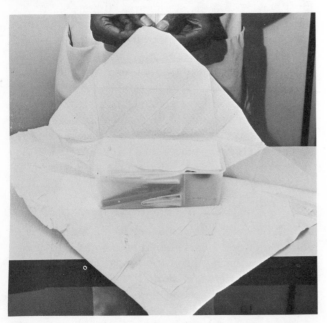

Figure 10-3

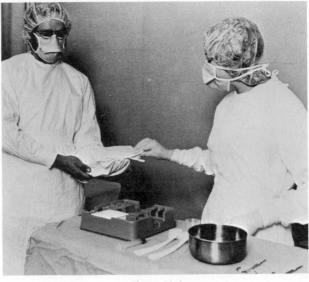

Figure 10-4

Opening Sterile Packs

The RT must be prepared to open sterile packs and either place them on the sterile field or hand them to the sterile person without contaminating the contents of the pack. There is a standard method for this procedure, which can be done without difficulty after it is practiced.

It is assumed that the RT has already washed his hands. When a request for a sterile item is received, the RT obtains the correct pack and returns it to the procedure room. A cloth-wrapped pack will be

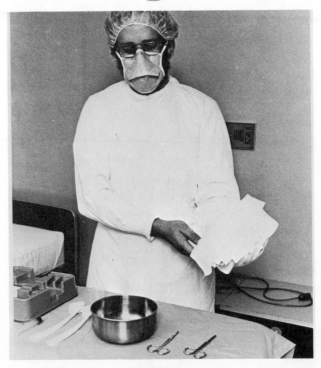

Figure 10-5

Central supply — sterile area
autoclaving is good for 3 months

sealed with indicator tape. The lines on the tape must be dark gray if the pack is sterile.

The pack is placed on a clean table top with the sealed end toward the RT. Remove the tape and discard it. Open corner one back and away from the pack (Fig. 10-1). Next, open corners two and three (Fig. 10-2). Then open corner four and drop it forward (Fig. 10-3). Do not touch the sterile contents of the pack. This can become a sterile field and more sterile items may be placed in the center of the drape, or the sterile contents of the pack can now be placed on another sterile field.

To do this, grasp the underside of the wrapper and let the edges fall over your hand. Hold the contents forward for the sterile person to grasp (Fig. 10-4). If it is preferable that the RT place the contents on the sterile field, he must grasp the corners of the wrapper with his other hand so that they do not brush the sterile field. He reaches slightly over the sterile field and several inches above it and drops the contents of the pack onto the field (Fig. 10-5).

Commercial packs are usually wrapped in paper or plastic containers. Directions for opening the container so there is no contamination are printed on the pack and should be read. The most common type of pack is sealed at the edges. The seal is separated at the top and peeled down until the sterile item is exposed. It can either be completely opened and made available for the sterile person to pick up, or it can be dropped onto the sterile field (Fig. 10-6).

A sterile forceps may be used to transfer objects from one sterile area to another. These forceps are usually large serrated ring forceps with ratchet closures. They are packaged in a sterile wrapper. The package should be opened so that there is a sterile surface on which to place the forceps when they are not in use. Only the tips are sterile.

When an object is to be transferred with a sterile forceps, the procedure is as follows. Open the sterile pack. Grasp the forceps by the handle, open the ratchet, and grasp the object to be transferred. Close the ratchet around the object. Transfer the object to the new location. Open the ratchet and drop the sterile object onto the sterile field. Replace the forceps on its sterile wrapper with the handles away from the center of the wrapper (Fig. 10-7).

The Surgical Scrub

Although the RT will rarely have occasion to be the sterile person in the operating room, it will benefit him to know the scrubbing procedure. For most purposes, the RT will have to change into a scrub suit and put on surgical shoe covers. The shoe covers are made of heavy paper and have a conductive strip

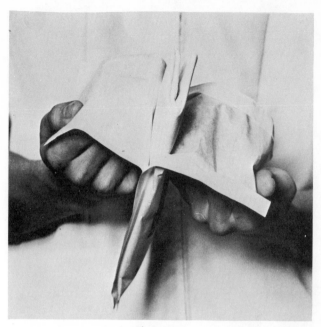

Figure 10-6

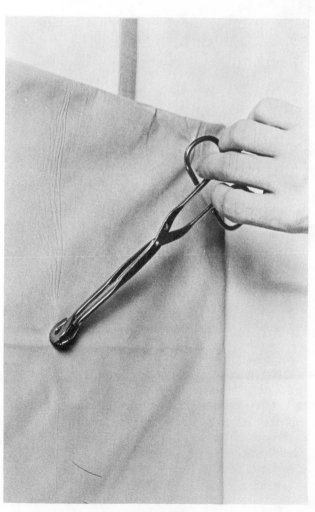

Figure 10-7

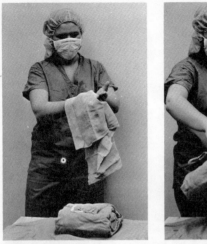

Figure 10-8

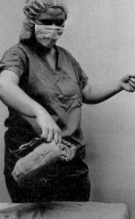

Figure 10-9

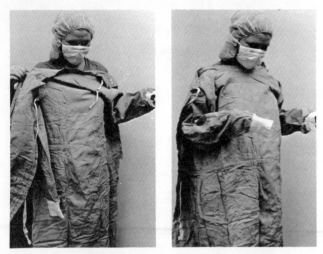

Figure 10-10

Figure 10-11

Figures 10-8 through 10-11 are from Eunice M. King, Lynn Wieck, and Marilyn Dyer, *Illustrated Manual of Nursing Techniques* (Philadelphia: J. B. Lippincott Company, 1977), p. 168.

built into them to prevent static electric sparks. Many hospital operating rooms no longer require these conduction devices because all of the equipment is grounded. The RT should follow hospital policy in this matter.

After donning surgical attire, the RT must place a surgical cap on his head so that his hair is completely covered. Remove all jewelry. Take a face mask out of the container. Handle the mask by the ties. Place the mask on so that it covers nose and mouth. Tie the mask at the back of the head and neck. Make certain that it is comfortable and secure. The mask must never be touched after it is in place, because it quickly becomes contaminated with microorganisms.

At this point the procedure will differ depending on the operating room assignment. If the RT

is to take radiographic exposures, he will scrub for three minutes. If he is to put on sterile gown and gloves, he must do a ten-minute surgical scrub. The procedure for this is as follows: The arms should be bare to at least 4 inches above the elbows.

1. Approach the scrub sink. Adjust the water temperature and pressure. Most surgical scrub areas have knee or foot regulators for the water faucets. If they do not, the faucet handles must be turned on, adjusted, and not touched again.
2. Wet hands and forearms to 2 inches above the elbows and apply surgical soap. Wash your hands according to the handwashing procedure described in Chapter 2. Rinse the soap off. The water should drain from the hands to the elbows or from the clean to the unclean area.
3. Obtain a nail cleaner and clean your nails under running water. Drop the nail cleaner into the sink.
4. Obtain a scrub brush from the dispenser and wet it. Re-wet hands and arms and re-apply soap.
5. Scrub hands, nails and the arms above the elbows using a firm, rotary motion. Rinse and repeat.
6. When finished, drop the brush into the sink. Proceed to the sterile area. Pick up a sterile towel by one corner. Drop it out in front of you at waist level. Do not let the towel touch your uniform. Dry one hand and arm with one end of the towel. Then use the other end to dry the other hand and arm (Fig. 10-8). Drop the towel to the floor. The RT will then proceed to the area where a sterile gown and gloves have been placed for him.

Sterile Gowning and Gloving

If the RT must open his own sterile gown and glove packs, this must be done before the surgical scrub. Usually an assistant is on hand to do this for the person who will be scrubbing. The sterile gown can be made of special paper or cloth. Grasp the gown and remove it from the table (Fig. 10-9). Step away from the table. The gown will be folded inside out. Hold the gown away from your body and allow it to unfold lengthwise without touching the floor. Open the gown and hold it by the shoulder seams. Place both arms in the arm holes and wait for assistance (Fig. 10-10). An assistant will approach the scrubbed person from behind, place his hands inside the gown at the shoulders and pull the gown over the shoulders and arms until the hands are bare (Fig. 10-11). The assistant then ties the gown at the neck and the waist, being careful to touch only the ties of the gown.

There are two methods of gloving for the operating room, the open and the closed. For the RT's purposes, the open method is the more practical and is the one that will be discussed.

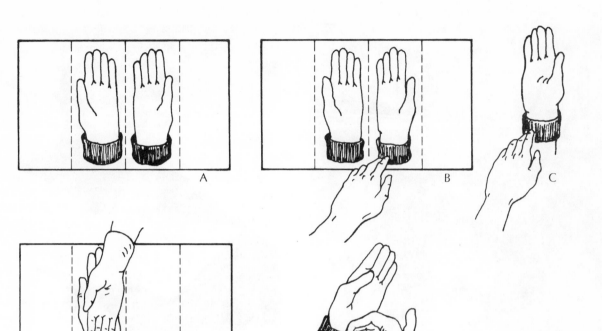

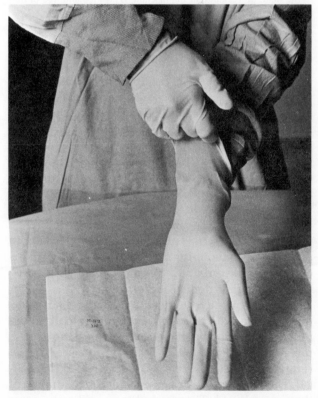

Figure 10-12.   From LuVerne Wolff Lewis, *Fundamental Skills in Patient Care* (Philadelphia: J. B. Lippincott Company, 1976), p. 296.

The glove wrapper is opened and the gloves are exposed. Sterile gloves are always folded down at the cuff and powdered so that they may be put on more easily (Fig. 10-12).

Pick up the right glove with the left hand at the folded cuff. Place the right hand in the glove, leaving the cuff of the glove folded down. When it is over the hand, leave it and pick up the left glove with the gloved right hand under the fold. Pull the glove over the hand and over the cuff of the gown in one motion (Fig. 10-13). Then place the fingers of the gloved left hand under the cuff of the right glove and pull it over the cuff of the gown. After the cuffs of the gloves cover the cuffs of the sterile gown, the gloves can be adjusted.

This procedure must be practiced several times before it is perfected. The RT must not be discouraged if he contaminates his gloves the first few times that he puts them on. The important thing is to notice when the gloves become contaminated and ask for another pair.

There are minor sterile procedures such as urinary catheterizations which require sterile gloves but not a sterile gown. If this is the case, the RT will wash his hands according to the rules of medical asepsis. Dry them well and then put on sterile gloves in the manner described.

Figure 10-13

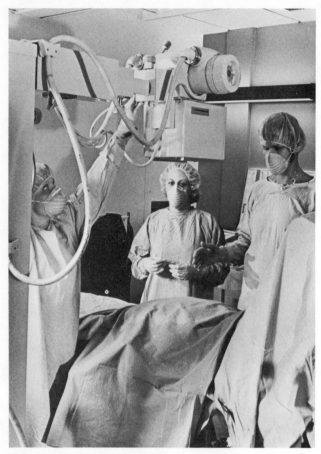

Figure 10-14. The portable machine is wheeled into place over the sterile field. Be certain that the machine is cleaned and free of dust before moving it into an operating room.

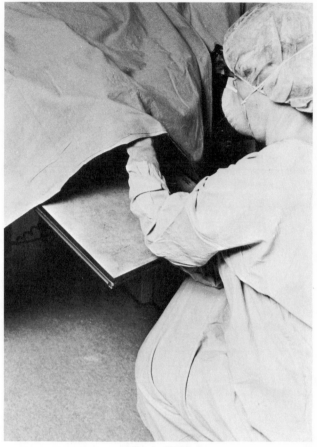

Figure 10-15

Radiographs in the Operating Room

When the RT is called to the operating room to make radiographic exposures, he must know what equipment the particular facility has for this purpose. In many modern hospitals the radiographic equipment remains in the operating suite at all times. This may not be the case in smaller hospitals, and the RT will have to transfer a portable radiographic machine from his department.

If he must do this, he will be responsible for cleaning it with an antiseptic solution before he changes into a scrub suit and before he scrubs in preparation for entering the operating suite with his equipment. Be certain that all equipment is prepared before changing clothes and scrubbing.

Frequently the need for a radiogram is anticipated, and the cassette may be put into place before the operation begins. At other times, the need is not anticipated and the RT will have to place his cassette after the sterile field has been created (Fig. 10-14). The RT must take care to prevent contamination of the surgical field. The surgical team will make room

for the RT, and he will have to approach the operating table and place the cassette. Do not touch the top side of the drape. Lift the drape from the underside only (Fig. 10-15). The RT who has a good knowledge of sterile technique will be comfortable in these situations and will be able to work with ease and efficiency.

Summary

The RT must participate in sterile procedures in the radiology department and in the operating suite. Any health worker who participates in sterile procedures must be strict in the practice of surgical asepsis, to prevent contamination and resulting infections.

The most common means of spreading microorganisms in the operating room is through use of contaminated instruments and gloves, by allowing a sterile field to become wet, and by failure to control air currents across sterile fields. All of these can be prevented by using good technique.

The best method of sterilizing surgical supplies and instruments is by steam under pressure (autoclaving). Other methods have proven to be unsatisfactory. Chemical agents may be used as disinfectants, but sterility is not ensured by their use. Before supplies are autoclaved, indicators of sterility are placed inside and outside the packs. These indicators change color or shape when the heat reaches peak temperature and indicate that sterilization is complete. The RT must learn to read the indicators used in his institution.

Before the RT begins to practice sterile technique, he must learn the rules of surgical asepsis. He must learn to differentiate sterile objects from unsterile objects. When there is doubt about the sterility of an object, it must be considered unsterile. The RT must learn the proper method of opening a sterile pack. An unsterile person must never reach across a sterile field. Any contamination of a sterile field must be remedied immediately.

A surgical scrub is a ten-minute scrub performed in the operating room before sterile gown and gloves are donned for a sterile procedure. The RT will not usually be the sterile person because he will be in the operating room only to make radiographic exposures. However, he must become familiar with operating room practices so that he can make these exposures without contaminating the surgical field. The RT who can practice good surgical asepsis is able to work more safely and efficiently.

See Appendix for pre-post test on Chapter 10.

Skin Preparation for Sterile Procedures

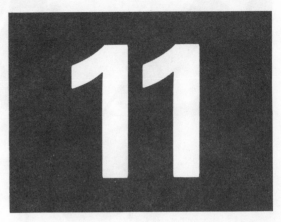

Many procedures done in the radiology department require special preparation of the skin. These procedures are all performed using sterile technique. The purpose of preparing the skin is to remove as many microorganisms as possible before the procedure is begun, because any procedure that involves penetration of the skin is apt to introduce microorganisms into the surgical wound. The RT may be called upon to perform this skin preparation, and he should be able to do it in the proper aseptic manner.

Occasionally the radiologist will request that a dressing be removed or re-applied. Surgical wounds must remain free of microorganisms. Draining "dirty" wounds are a potential source of contamination for the RT and for others in the department. The RT must be able to remove or re-apply a dressing using aseptic technique to protect the patient and himself and others from contamination.

Skin Preparation for Sterile Procedures

Both mechanical and chemical methods are used to prepare the skin prior to a procedure which involves surgical penetration of the skin. They are followed by draping the skin with sterile materials.

The mechanical method of skin preparation includes the removal of hair as necessary and the cleansing of the skin with soap and water.

Chemical preparation involves the application of an antiseptic to kill microorganisms remaining on the skin. Sterile drapes are then applied around the

Goal of This Chapter
The RT will learn to prepare the patient's skin for sterile procedures and to change dressings in an aseptic manner.

Objectives
When the student has completed this chapter, he will be able to:
1. Prepare the skin for a sterile procedure in the radiology department.
2. Demonstrate, in the laboratory, the correct method of removing and re-applying a dressing.

Glossary
Betadine   a proprietary name for a preparation of povidone-iodine, an antiseptic

fenestrated   having one or more openings

pHisoHex   a proprietary name for an emulsion containing hexachlorophene (an antiseptic detergent)

Zephiran   a proprietary name for a preparation of benzalkonium chloride, an antiseptic

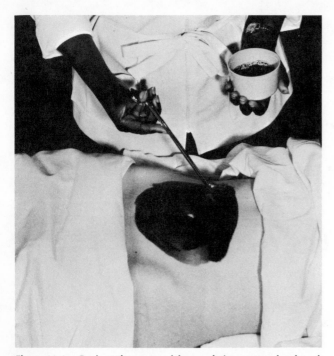

Figure 11-1.   Begin at the center of the area being prepared and work outward in a circular motion.

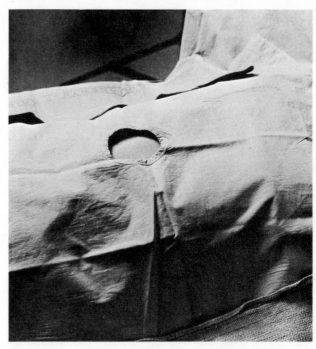

Figure 11-2

prepared area of the skin to protect it from outside contamination.

After the patient is positioned for a special procedure, the hair on his skin should be examined. Before any hair is shaved, the radiologist must state that it is to be done. If it is ordered, the RT should wash his hands and obtain a prep set, which includes a basin, a sponge, a razor, a towel, and soap. Explain to the patient what must be done and place him in a comfortable position.

Fill the basin with warm water. Wet the sponge and apply soap. For this purpose pHisoHex is often used. Wet the patient's skin in the area to be shaved and soap it. Remove the hair with short, firm strokes. Hold the skin taut and shave in the direction of the hair growth.

After the hair has been removed, clean the skin well with warm water and soap. The area cleansed should always extend at least 6 inches beyond the area to be penetrated in each direction.

When all necessary shaving and cleansing of the skin is complete, the skin is painted with an antiseptic solution. The solution used varies, but Betadine and Zephiran solutions are acceptable in most hospitals.

The RT will need a sterile forceps, sterile cotton balls or gauze sponges, and a small sterile medicine glass or metal cup in which to pour the antiseptic.

Pick up the sterile gauze sponges or cotton balls with the sterile forceps and dip them into the

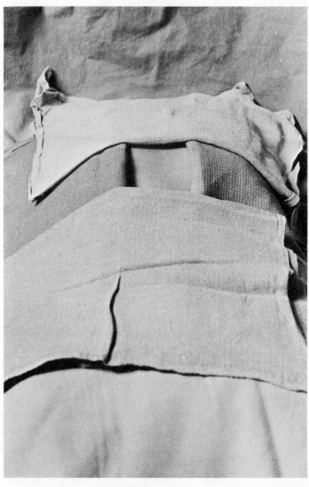

Figure 11-3

solution. Begin the prep at the center of the area and work in a circular pattern to the outer edges of the area. Drop the used sponge into the container prepared for this purpose. Wait for the antiseptic to dry and repeat the procedure (Fig. 11-1).

Draping for Sterile Procedures

After the skin has been mechanically and chemically prepared and allowed to dry, sterile drapes may be applied. They are placed around the area of skin that has been prepared. The type of sterile drape differs with each procedure. In the radiology department, usually the drape will be a paper one, and it may be fenestrated. If this is the case, the drape should be applied in such a way that the opening leaves only the operative site exposed (Fig. 11-2). If sterile towels are used, they should be placed so that they are well within the limits of the area prepared and should overlap. Cloth drapes should be of double thickness (Fig. 11-3).

Often the radiologist places the sterile drapes after he has donned sterile gloves for the procedure, so the RT must have the sterile pack that contains the drapes open and ready for him. Many pre-packaged procedure sets contain sterile drapes.

If the RT is to place the sterile drapes, he must first open a set of sterile gloves for himself. Then the pack containing the drapes is opened. The sterile gloves are then donned and the drapes are placed. Once a drape is in place, it may not be moved because the underside is now contaminated and moving it will contaminate the operative area. The RT must protect his gloves as he applies sterile drapes by cuffing the drape around his gloved hands.

Dressing Change

The RT must not remove dressings or reapply them unless it is requested by the physician. When the physician requests that a dressing be removed for a procedure in the radiology department, the RT must be able to remove it without contaminating the wound or himself in the process.

All dressings must be treated as if they were contaminated, because draining wounds often harbor staphylococci. When you remove a dressing, obtain a sterile forceps and a waterproof paper bag or paper towels onto which the soiled dressing will be placed. Dressings should not be touched with bare hands. If no forceps is available, obtain sterile gloves and don them after everything is in readiness for removal of the dressing.

Wash your hands. Place the patient in a comfortable position and explain what you are going to do. Loosen the adhesive tape that holds the dressing

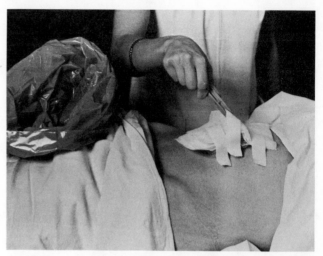

Figure 11-4

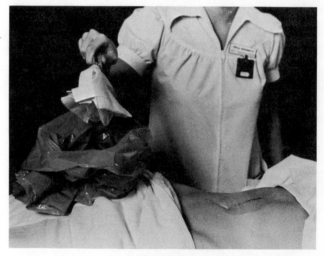

Figure 11-5

in place. This is painful and must be done with care. Remove the dressing carefully with a forceps or gloved hands and place it into the paper receptacle. Wrap the soiled dressing completely and dispose of it properly (Figs. 11-4 and 11-5). If the dressing does not come off easily, stop the procedure and report this to the radiologist. Never use force to remove a dressing, as this may cause further damage to a wound or cause the wound to bleed. When the dressing is removed, remove the gloves and dispose of them or place the soiled forceps in the area kept for soiled instruments. Wash your hands.

When a dressing is re-applied, sterile technique must always be used. Wash your hands and obtain the necessary equipment. You will need a sterile towel, gauze pads, tape, a paper bag or receptacle for refuse, and sterile gloves. Occasionally a sterile pad large enough to cover the abdomen will be needed to be applied over the small gauze pad if the wound is draining.

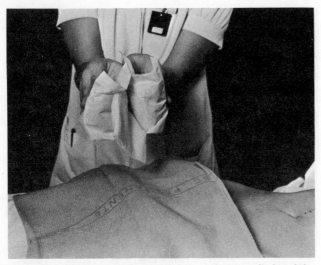

Figure 11-6. When an abdominal dressing is being applied, and the patient is cooperative, the sterile towel may be placed below the abdominal wound.

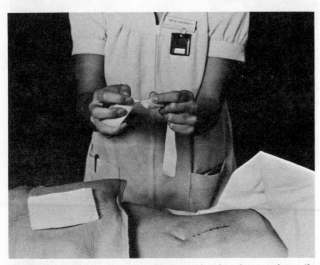

Figure 11-7. The tape is not sterile. It must be placed so as to be easily retrieved, but not on the sterile field.

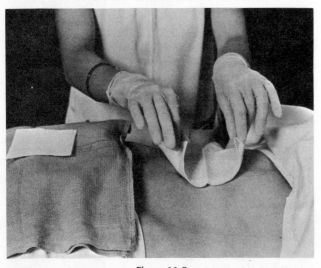

Figure 11-8

When the materials are ready, approach the patient and explain the procedure to him. If the dressing has not been removed, remove it in the manner just described.

Open the sterile towel and use it as a sterile field on which to place sterile dressings. Open the dressings and place them on the sterile towel (Fig. 11-6). Prepare the tape and have it cut into proper lengths (Fig. 11-7). Put on the sterile gloves. Apply the dressing, remove the gloves, and secure the dressing with tape (Fig. 11-8). Wash your hands and properly dispose of waste materials. Make the patient comfortable.

Summary

The skin is prepared for any surgical penetration to remove as many microorganisms as possible from the operative site. This reduces the possibility of infection from the procedure. Mechanical and chemical methods are used to prepare the skin, followed by application of sterile drapes around the surgical area.

The RT may be required to remove or re-apply a dressing to a wound. These procedures should be done using aseptic technique. Any dressing that is removed must be considered to harbor pathogenic microorganisms. Soiled dressings must not be touched with bare hands. Gloves or forceps must be used. The soiled dressing must be wrapped in a waterproof bag or double thickness of paper towels and disposed of properly.

When dressings are removed or re-applied, the patient must be protected from infection. The RT must also protect himself and others in his department. Use of aseptic technique and proper disposal of waste materials will accomplish this.

See Appendix for pre-post test on Chapter 11.

Catheterization of the Urinary Bladder and Catheter Care

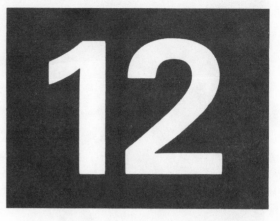

Catheterization of the urinary bladder refers to the introduction of a plastic or rubber tube through the urethra into the bladder. This is part of many examinations done in the radiology department. It is important for the RT to learn the correct method of catheterizing so that he may properly insert a catheter or assist with insertion of a catheter.

Some medical reasons for use of catheters are the following: to keep the urinary bladder empty while the tissues around it heal for patients who have had operative procedures that require this; to provide for drainage, irrigation, or instillation of chemotherapeutic solutions into the bladder; and to assist incontinent patients to control urinary flow. These patients will come to the radiology department with retention or Foley catheters in place.

Two of the examinations performed in the radiology department that involve insertion of a catheter are cystourethrograms and cystograms.

The urinary bladder is sterile; any object or solution that is placed in the bladder must be sterile. Use of improper technique when performing catheterization of the urinary bladder or when caring for a patient who has a retention catheter in place may cause infection. Injury to the patient is also possible during this procedure. Urinary catheterization is never performed without a specific order by the physician. Because of the hazards of injury and infection, the RT must never perform this procedure by himself until he has been adequately supervised and is certain of the technique required. Most hospitals

Goal of This Chapter
The RT student will learn to insert a catheter into the urinary bladder and to care for patients who have Foley catheters in place.

Objectives
When the student has completed this chapter, he will be able to:
1. Demonstrate, in the laboratory, the correct method of inserting a French or Foley catheter into the urinary bladder.
2. Explain, in writing, the proper method of transporting a patient who has a Foley catheter in place.
3. Give a written explanation of the three most important considerations in caring for a patient who has an indwelling catheter.

Glossary
Foley catheter an indwelling urinary catheter with an inflatable balloon that holds it in position

glans the cap-shaped expansion of the corpus spongiosum at the end of the penis

meatus a general term for a passageway to the body (urinary meatus)

perineum the pelvic floor and the associated structures occupying the pelvic outlet, bounded anteriorly by the symphysis pubis; laterally by the ischial tuberosities and posteriorly by the coccyx

sphincter a ringlike band of muscle fiber that constricts a passage or closes a natural orifice

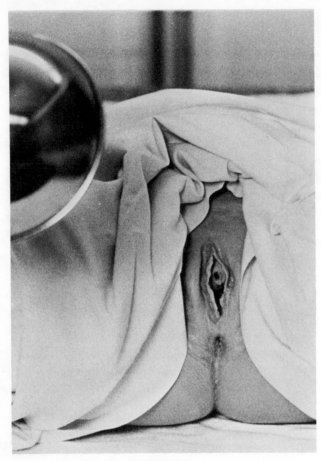

Figure 12-1

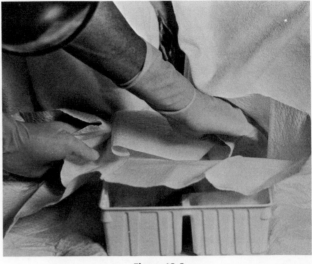

Figure 12-2

prefer that male nurses or technologists catheterize male patients and female nurses or technologists catheterize females.

Female Catheterization

When the RT has been requested to catheterize a patient, he must establish whether the physician desires to use a retention (Foley) catheter or a straight French catheter. Most hospitals provide prepared trays for this purpose, with the desired type of catheter included.

The equipment needed to perform a catheterization is as follows: a French or Foley catheter, antiseptic solution, cotton balls for cleansing, water-soluble lubricant, a specimen bottle, a receptacle for waste urine, sterile drapes, forceps, and sterile gloves. A prepared tray will include all of these items. A drape sheet and a goose neck lamp are necessary for catheterization of a female patient. Do not attempt to catheterize a female unless adequate lighting is provided.

After the equipment has been assembled, wash your hands. Approach the patient and identify her. Explain what must be done. Patients are often

embarrassed and apprehensive about this procedure. A good explanation and reassurance that there will be little, if any, pain are important. Tell the patient that there will be a slight sensation of pressure when the catheter is inserted. Provide privacy for the patient, and, if possible, use a screen, or close the door to the procedure room.

Drape the patient with a sheet or cotton blanket from the waist down. Place the patient on her back, then have her flex her knees and drop them apart as far as she can. Drape the sheet so that only the perineum is exposed. If a patient is disabled and cannot maintain this position, the RT may need an assistant to maintain adequate exposure. Adjust the light so that it shines directly on the perineal area. It is difficult to locate the meatus in many females unless adequate lighting is available (Fig. 12-1).

Open the sterile pack which has been placed between the patient's legs. The gloves will be the top-most item and they will be cuffed for ease in donning. The sterile drapes are just under the gloves. When you have donned the sterile gloves, pick up the first drape. Cover your gloves with the drape to protect them from contamination. Place the first drape under the patient's hips (Fig. 12-2). A fenestrated drape may be placed over the perineal area. Pour antiseptic solution over the cotton balls. Open the lubricant package and squeeze some of it out onto the sterile drape.

With the left hand, separate the labia minora until the meatus is clearly visible. This glove is now contaminated and will be used only to maintain exposure. Pick up one cotton ball with the small forceps and cleanse the far side of the meatus with a single downward stroke. Drop the cotton ball and pick up another. Wipe the near side of the meatus with a

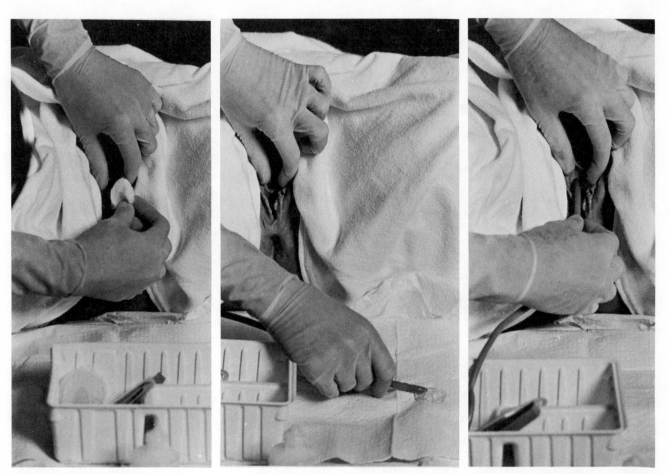

Figure 12-3   Figure 12-4   Figure 12-5

single downward stroke. With the third cotton ball, cleanse directly over the meatus with a single downward stroke (Fig. 12-3). Keep the left hand in place to maintain exposure. With the right hand, pick up the catheter 1 inch from the tip. Lubricate it with the sterile lubricant that was placed on the sterile drape (Fig. 12-4). Then slowly insert the catheter into the meatus (Fig. 12-5). If there is any resistance, do not continue the procedure. The catheter will usually pass unobstructed into the bladder. When urine begins to flow out of the catheter, it has passed through the sphincter and into the bladder.

If a French catheter is being employed, place the drainage basin under the distal end of the catheter to catch the urine and allow it to drain; if a Foley catheter, a drainage bag may be attached at the end, and the urine will flow into it. The inflatable balloon will be inflated after the catheter is in the bladder. It is most often filled with 5 cc. of sterile distilled water (Fig. 12-6).

Often, the catheterization set will include a syringe previously filled with water and placed on the valve of the catheter. If not, draw up 5 cc. of sterile distilled water and attach it to the catheter valve. Push

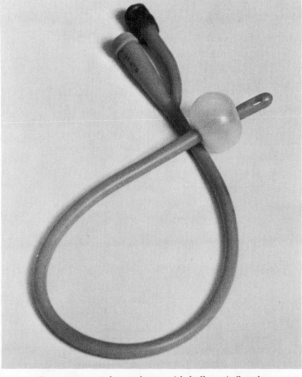

Figure 12-6.   Foley catheter with balloon inflated.

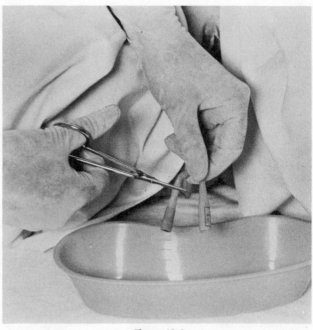

Figure 12-9

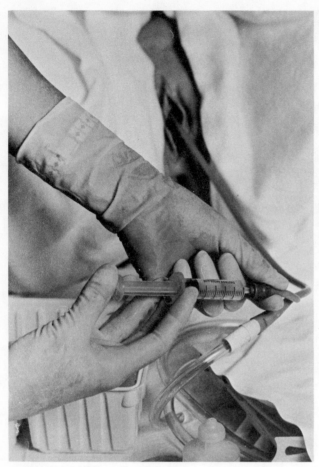

Figure 12-7

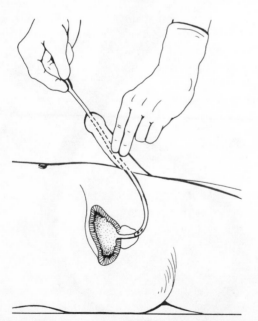

Figure 12-8. From LuVerne Wolff Lewis, *Fundamental Skills in Patient Care* (Philadelphia: J. B. Lippincott Company, 1976), p. 313.

the plunger of the syringe down to inflate the balloon. Most catheter valves are self-sealing. When the syringe is withdrawn, the procedure is completed (Fig. 12-7). Gently pull on the catheter to be certain that it will be retained. If there is resistance, the balloon is properly inflated.

Remove the soiled equipment and make the patient comfortable. Remove your gloves. If the catheter is to remain in the patient for some time, it should be taped to the inner thigh to prevent it from becoming dislodged. Arrangements should be made for urinary drainage depending upon the procedure that is to follow.

Male Catheterization

The equipment needed is the same as for female catheterization, though a slightly larger catheter may be required. The patient is placed in the supine position. Open the sterile pack at the patient's proximal side. Drape the patient with one sterile drape above the genital area and another under the penis.

Follow the same procedure as for female catheterization. Grasp the penis firmly and spread the urinary meatus between the thumb and forefinger. If the penis is not handled firmly an erection may be stimulated. Cleanse the glans using a circular motion. Drop the cotton ball. Next, cleanse directly over the meatus. Discard the cotton ball.

Lubricate the catheter, holding it about 4 inches from the tip. Draw the penis forward and up-

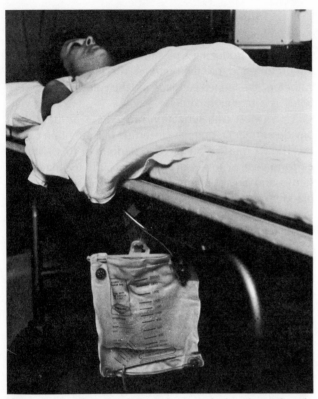

Figure 12-10.   The urine drainage bag must be kept lower than the level of the bladder when a patient with a Foley catheter in place is being transported.

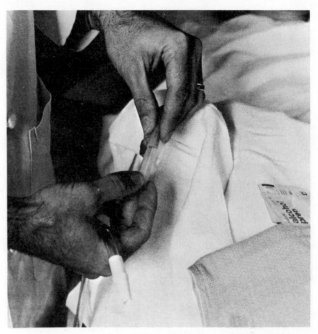

Figure 12-11.   Insert a sterile plug into the Foley catheter.

should come out easily and with no resistance. When it is completely removed, fold paper towels around it. Remove the soiled equipment and cover the patient. Most catheters are disposable and are discarded. Catheters are rarely sterilized for re-use.

Catheter Care in the Radiology Department

Often patients must be transported to the radiology department with retention catheters in place. If this is the case, the RT must keep the drainage bag below the level of the bladder so that the gravity flow is maintained. If urine is allowed to flow back into the bladder, or if the drainage is obstructed, infection may result (Fig. 12-10).

Care must be taken when moving a patient with a catheter in place to avoid undue tension being placed on the catheter. This can cause the patient great discomfort or injury, if it becomes dislodged.

Occasionally it is necessary to disconnect a catheter from its drainage bag. This must never be done without an order from the physician. If it is to be done, great care must be taken to keep the end of the catheter and the end of the tubing sterile. A sterile plug and cap set should be obtained. The area where the catheter is to be disconnected should be cleaned with antiseptic solution. Then, using aseptic technique, place the sterile plug into the catheter and the sterile cover over the end of the drainage tubing (Figs. 12-11 and 12-12).

ward, stretching it slightly. Ask the patient to try to void as this will relax the sphincter. Using gentle constant pressure, insert the catheter (Fig. 12-8). Too much force may cause a spasm of the sphincter and delay insertion. Do not try to proceed if there is an obstruction. Withdraw the catheter and notify the physician. When there is a flow of urine, the catheter is in the bladder. At this time, the balloon will be inflated if the catheter is a retention type.

Secure the catheter with tape if necessary. Make the patient comfortable and wash your hands.

Removing a Foley Catheter

To remove an indwelling catheter, you will need a scissors, a small basin (an emesis basin will do), and several paper towels.

Wash your hands, identify the patient, and explain the procedure. Uncover the patient enough to expose the catheter. Place the collecting basin under the valve of the catheter. Cut the tip of the valve off and allow the water to drain into the basin (Fig. 12-9). When the flow of water stops, place the paper towels under the catheter and gently pull it out. If there is resistance, do not continue to pull. The catheter

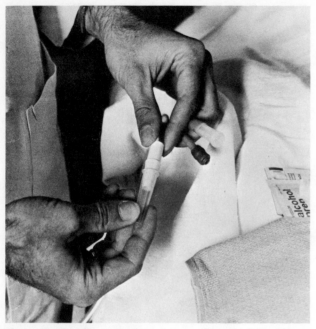

Figure 12-12. Place a sterile cover over the end of the drainage tubing if it is to be re-used.

A catheter must not remain clamped for longer than one hour, and there are occasions when this may be too long to leave a catheter clamped. If the patient complains of pressure in the area of his urinary bladder or of a need to urinate, the catheter must be reconnected to its drainage bag, again with use of aseptic technique. If the procedure being done prevents this, the radiologist must be notified of the patient's complaint.

Summary

Catheterization of the urinary bladder is the process of introducing a plastic or rubber tubing through the urethra and into the bladder. There are two types of catheters, the French catheter and the Foley catheter. The Foley is a retention catheter.

Most catheterization procedures in the radiology department require the insertion of a retention catheter. The RT must be prepared to perform or to assist with performance of this procedure. The urinary bladder is sterile and any solution or object introduced into the bladder must be sterile.

The same type of equipment is required for catheterization of both males and females, though the procedure varies slightly due to anatomical differences. Usually a male RT will catheterize male patients and a female RT will catheterize female patients. The patient must be given proper explanation, reassurance, and privacy before the procedure is begun.

Proper care of retention catheters while patients are being transported to the radiology department, or are being cared for there, must not be forgotten. The RT must be certain that the drainage bag remains below the level of the bladder to ensure proper gravity flow of urine. Tension on the catheter should be avoided. If a catheter is clamped, or disconnected, aseptic technique must be followed. A catheter should not be clamped without orders from the physician. It must not remain clamped for more than one hour. If the patient complains of pain or pressure within less than one hour, the catheter must be unclamped and allowed to drain.

See Appendix for pre-post test on chapter 12.

Assisting with Drug Administration

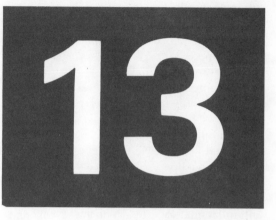

13

Goal of This Chapter
The RT student will learn to assist with administration of drugs orally and parenterally with safety and accuracy.

Objectives
When the student has completed this chapter, he will be able to:
1. List three precautions necessary when assisting with drug administration.
2. List five physical factors that influence drug action.
3. List five methods of drug administration.
4. Demonstrate in the laboratory and in writing the proper equipment needed to administer any drug requested by the physician.
5. Define the basic prescription abbreviations commonly used in hospitals.
6. List the anatomical sites most commonly used when administering parenteral medications by intravenous, subcutaneous, intramuscular, and intradermal routes.
7. List three physical symptoms that indicate a problem with an intravenous infusion.
8. Describe two complaints that can develop in a patient who is experiencing an adverse drug reaction.
9. Define the terminology that describes drug actions.

Glossary
acidosis a disturbance in the acid-base balance of the body causing an increase in acids

addictive causing physical dependence

adsorbent a substance that causes other substances to adhere to its surface

adverse acting against or in a contrary direction

The RT must not administer medications. He is not trained or licensed to do so. A violation of this restriction is professional malpractice. However, the RT will be asked to assist with drug administration in the radiology department, and he must be a safe and competent assistant. Any drug administered by any route is potentially hazardous. Frequently the RT will be the only observer of the patient after a drug has been administered. As a professional person, he must familiarize himself with the safety measures to be taken when drugs are being given. He must also be an accurate observer and be able to detect symptoms of adverse reactions to drugs in order to take the correct action if these reactions occur. Rapid detection of adverse drug reactions is often of utmost importance if the patient's life is to be saved.

Drug Classifications

Drugs may be classified in several ways. For convenience, in this chapter, they will be classified according to their action on various parts of the body. The same drug may be sold under many different proprietary or trade names. The trade name is the name assigned to a drug by a particular manufacturer, and the same drug may be manufactured by another company and given a different proprietary name. The trade name of a drug is copyrighted and cannot be used by another manufacturer.

The chemical name of a drug represents its exact chemical formula. This remains the same always. A drug's generic name, like the chemical name,

Glossary cont.

agranulocytosis   a disease in which the white blood cell count drops to a very low level and an abnormally small number of neutrophil cells are present in the blood

alopecia   an abnormal baldness that may be spotty or complete

analgesic   drug used to relieve pain

antacid   substance that counteracts or neutralizes gastrointestinal acidity

antifungal   destructive to fungi or suppressing their reproduction

antihistamine   a drug that counteracts the action of histamine

anti-inflammatory   an agent that counteracts or suppresses inflammation

antipruritic   a drug that relieves itching

antipyretic   an agent that decreases body temperature

aplastic anemia   a disease that results in reduction in the number of circulating red blood cells due to failure of production of bone marrow

apothecaries measure   the series of units of liquid measure (such as the gallon, pint, fluid ounce, and minim)

aqueous solution   solution having a water base or a watery base

arthralgia   joint pain

aspiration   the act of inhaling; the removal of fluids or gases from a cavity by the application of suction

astringent   agent or substance that inhibits secretions from wounds or mucous membranes, stops bleeding, lessens peristalsis, or hardens tissues

autonomic nervous system   that part of the nervous system concerned with regulating the activity of cardiac muscle, smooth muscles, and glands

blanched   colorless, white, or pale

buccal   pertaining to the inside of the cheek

cardiovascular system   the heart and blood vessels, by which the blood is circulated throughout the body

carminative   a medicine that relieves flatulence (gas) and cramping in the digestive tract

catalyst   a substance which speeds up the rate of chemical action

central nervous system   that part of the nervous system that consists of the brain and the spinal cord

ciliary muscle   muscle that controls certain structures of the eye

cretinism   a congenital state characterized by lack of physical and mental development

demulcent   an agent that soothes or softens skin on surfaces where applied

depressant   agent that temporarily decreases activity of a body function (cardiac, respiratory)

derivative   a chemical substance derived from another substance either directly, by modification, or by partial substitution

dermatitis   an inflammation of the skin with symptoms such as itching, redness, and rash

digestant   an agent that stimulates or assists in digestion

diuretic   a drug that increases the flow of urine

dorsal   pertaining to the back

dyspnea   air hunger

emetic   an agent that induces vomiting

enzyme   a protein capable of accelerating or producing by catalytic action some change in a basic substance

fluid intoxication   state of being poisoned by an excessive intake of fluid

habituating   becoming accustomed to by frequent use; not a physical dependence as in addiction

hallucination   a false perception not caused by external stimuli; may be auditory or visual

hematoma   a tumor or swelling which contains blood

hemochromatosis   a disorder of iron metabolism characterized by iron deposits in the tissues, especially of the liver, kidneys, and pancreas, and a bronze pigmentation of the skin

household measure   measurement with cup, teaspoon, and so on

hyperkinesia   abnormally increased motor function or activity

hypertension   persistently high arterial blood pressure

hypertonic   a solution having increased tonicity or tension

hypothyroidism   a condition due to a deficiency of thyroid secretion

inhalation   the drawing of air or other substances into the lung

intraocular   within the eyeball

lactation   the function of secreting milk

libido   the sexual drive, conscious or unconscious

lumen   the space within a tube

metric system   a system of measurement based on the meter

multisynaptic   many points of contact

myxedema   swelling due to low-functioning thyroid gland

neuralgia   severe sharp pain along the course of a nerve

oral   by mouth

osteoporosis   increased porousness of bones

parasiticide   an agent that is destructive to parasites

parasympathetic   the craniosacral portion of the autonomic nervous system

Parkinson's disease   a group of neurological disorders characterized by hypokinesia, tremors, and muscular rigidity

pediculosis   infestation with lice

Glossary cont.

peripheral   situated away from the center of a structure

precipitate   a deposit made or a substance thrown down by precipitation

pulmonary edema   the presence of abnormally large amounts of fluid in the lungs

scabies   a highly communicable skin disease caused by the itch mite

sedative   a drug which lessens the activity of an organ of the body, or decreases nervous excitability

stimulant   a drug that temporarily increases functional activity

sublingual   under the tongue

sympathetic nervous system   the portion of the autonomic nervous system that plays a role in the excitation and relaxation of muscles and provides an important additional surface for the exchange of substances produced by metabolism between muscle and the extracellular spaces

tachycardia   abnormally rapid heart action

tetany   a nervous affliction which results in intermittent contractions or spasms usually of the extremities

therapeutic   having the ability to cure

thrombus   a blood clot that obstructs a blood vessel

vasodilatation   dilatation of a vessel

---

is not the property of any particular company. It is a drug's distinctive name and remains unchanged. The RT must be aware that any drug used in his department may be represented by several trade names. If he checks the generic name, which is always listed on the label under the trade name, he will be able to identify the drug, regardless of which proprietary name is used.

In the lists that follow, the RT will find a description of drug categories, the major drugs in each category, the purpose for which each drug is administered, and the route of administration. In a text such as this one, it is not possible to list every drug in each category. The aim is to acquaint the RT with those drugs which he is likely to encounter in his work.

ANTIBIOTICS

These drugs inhibit growth of bacteria or kill bacteria. They are manufactured from substances produced by specific fungi. Most antibiotics are effective against rapidly multiplying microorganisms. Some are more effective against gram-positive microorganisms, some against gram-negative microorganisms. The broad-spectrum antibiotics are effective against both.

MAJOR DRUGS (PROPRIETARY NAME IN PARENTHESES)	PURPOSE	ROUTE OF ADMINISTRATION	ADVERSE EFFECTS
Penicillins	Chiefly effective against gram-positive and certain gram-negative microorganisms including meningococcus (meningitis) and gonococcus (gonorrhea)	Oral or parenteral	Generally non-toxic; but observe patient for allergic reaction, such as rash, edema, other symptoms of allergy
Streptomycin	Active against several gram-negative and limited number of gram-positive microorganisms including tubercle bacillus (tuberculosis)	Usually intramuscular injection; occasionally oral or by nebulizer	Rare when used for only few days; more frequent whzn used for long periods; reactions include dizziness, ringing in ears, disturbances in equilibrium, hearing deficiencies; also headache, nausea, vomiting, rash
Chloramphenicol (Chloromycetin) Tetracyclines	Effective against greater numbers of gram-positive and gram-negative microorganisms	Oral	Relatively non-toxic; but nausea, vomiting, diarrhea may occur; chloramphenicol has caused depression in production of bone marrow, with development of aplastic anemia and agranulocytosis, consequently use of this drug has been sharply reduced

DRUGS THAT ACT ON THE AUTONOMIC NERVOUS SYSTEM

The autonomic nervous system has two divisions, the sympathetic and the parasympathetic divisions. Drugs are employed selectively to stimulate or depress the function of these divisions in order to regulate heart rate, vasoconstriction or dilation, gastrointestinal function, the energy requirements of the body, ciliary muscle of the eye, the urinary bladder, and the salivary and lacrimal glands.

MAJOR DRUGS (PROPRIETARY NAME IN PARENTHESES)	PURPOSE	ROUTE OF ADMINISTRATION	ADVERSE EFFECTS
Epinephrine* (Adrenalin)	Diverts blood flow from skin and mucous membranes to brain, liver, heart, skeletal muscles, thereby increasing heartbeat; constricts arterioles of skin, mucous membranes, lungs, kidneys	Parenteral; sometimes by local application	Toxicity, ranging from anxiety, nervousness, pallor to cardiac arrhythmias and circulatory collapse
Metaraminol bitartrate (Aramine)*	Strong vasoconstricting drug, used to elevate blood pressure	Parenteral; topical (as nasal decongestant)	Dangerously elevated blood pressure
Nicotine	Vasoconstrictor; stimulates sympathetic nervous system; not widely used medically	(Not used medically.)	Toxic in large doses; forbidden for patients with cardiovascular disease
Atropine sulfate	Synthetic alkaloid of belladonna; used locally to paralyze muscles of light accommodation in eye; decreases secretions of nose, pharynx, bronchial tubes; produces relaxation of bronchi, thus dilating airway to ease breathing; accelerates heart action by interfering with cardiac response to vagal nerve impulses; reduces or stops sweat gland activity, thus causing skin to become hot and dry	Oral, parenteral, or topical (as ophthalmic solution)	Mild reactions include thirst, difficult swallowing, flushed face, elevated body temperature; severe toxic reactions: staggering gait, stupor, coma, respiratory or circulatory failure; should not be given to patients with glaucoma or increased intraocular pressure

* Found on every emergency drug tray.

DRUGS THAT ACT ON THE CENTRAL NERVOUS SYSTEM

These drugs include central nervous system stimulants; drugs that affect behavior; drugs that depress the central nervous system; drugs used to control hyperkinesia, epilepsy, skeletal muscle spasm, and Parkinson's disease; and drugs used to treat motion sickness and nausea.

MAJOR DRUGS (PROPRIETARY NAME IN PARENTHESES)	PURPOSE	ROUTE OF ADMINISTRATION	ADVERSE EFFECTS
Aminophylline*	Dilates bronchioles; useful in treatment of acute asthmatic symptoms, respiratory distress	Intravenous; oral; rectal suppository	Bronchospasm, nausea may occur
Chlorpromazine hydrochloride (Thorazine)	Tranquilizing drug used to control anxiety, tension, hyperactive behavior in psychotic and neurotic patients; controls nausea; used as a preoperative medication in combination with narcotics to potentiate their action	Oral; parenteral	Prolonged use may cause jaundice due to liver damage; restlessness, tremors, shuffling gait, blood dyscrasias; immediate reactions include subnormal blood pressure, dermatitis
Promethazine hydrochloride (Phenergan)	Similar to above; also potent antihistamine	Oral; parenteral; rectal	Dryness of mouth, blurred vision; should not be used with alcohol

DRUGS THAT ACT ON THE CENTRAL NERVOUS SYSTEM cont.

MAJOR DRUGS (PROPRIETARY NAME IN PARENTHESES)	PURPOSE	ROUTE OF ADMINISTRATION	ADVERSE EFFECTS
Meprobamate Chlordiazepoxide Diazepam (Valium)	Muscle relaxants; relieve anxiety, tension; promote rest, sleep; used in treatment of alcoholism and neuroses	Oral; parenteral	Rash, nausea, dizziness, drug dependence; overdose will cause falling blood pressure, coma; decreased tolerance to alcohol so should not be used with alcohol
Morphine	Analgesic	Parenteral	Addictive; respiratory depression, hypotension, constipation, skin rash
Codeine	Analgesic; relieves mild pain; cough suppressant	Oral; parenteral	Addictive; dryness of mouth; convulsions likely to occur if administered to children
Meperidine hydrochloride (Demerol)	Synthetic used in place of morphine as is less potent; has slight sedative effect; analgesic	Oral; parenteral	Addictive; dizziness, nausea, respiratory depression, decreased blood pressure
Acetylsalicylic acid (aspirin) Acetaminophen (Tylenol)	Mild analgesics; antipyretic effect; commonly used for headache, neuralgia, arthralgia, fever	Oral	Prolonged use may cause gastric bleeding, ringing in ears, rash, dizziness, hearing disturbances; overdose may cause poisoning with symptoms of depression, circulatory collapse, respiratory failure
Phenobarbital Sodium secobarbital (Seconal) Sodium pentobarbital (Nembutal)	Barbiturates; sedative effect; depending on dose, may range from mild sedation to hypnosis to general anesthesia	Oral; some parenteral	Prolonged use of small doses can cause dependency; prolonged use of large doses, addiction; restlessness, excitement, hallucinations; overdosage causes respiratory depression and peripheral collapse
Chloral hydrate	Synthetic sedative hypnotic used occasionally as pretreatment medication in radiology department	Oral	Relatively safe; respiratory depression; prolonged use may result in habituation
Sodium diphenylhydantoin** (Dilantin)	Barbiturate; controls convulsive seizures as inhibits spread of abnormal impulses in motor cortex of brain without decreasing mental activity	Oral; parenteral	Rash, dizziness, nervousness, blurred vision, soreness and bleeding of gums, hallucinations, nausea
Methocarbamol (Robaxin)	Relaxes skeletal muscles by suppressing multisynaptic reflexes of spinal cord	Oral; parenteral	Dizziness, drowsiness, headache, blurred vision, rash, nausea
Cyclizine hydrochloride (Marezine) Dimenhydrinate (Dramamine)	Used to treat motion sickness and nausea	Oral; parenteral	Drowsiness, dry mouth, blurred vision
Ethyl alcohol (also known as ethanol)	Used as vasodilator in peripheral vascular disease to improve appetite and digestion; to induce sleep; inhibits contractions at onset of premature labor when used in form of intravenous drip	Oral; parenteral	Excitement, depression, stupor, depressed respirations; may be addictive
Amphetamine Dexamphetamine sulfate (Dexedrine Sulfate)	Central nervous system stimulants; increase mental alertness, elevate spirits, reduce fatigue; depress appetite, reduce drowsiness	Oral	Increased nervousness, excitability, hypertension; overdose can cause chills, rapid heartbeat, collapse; may be habituating (Dexamphetamine sulfate does not cause hypertension)

DRUGS THAT ACT ON THE CENTRAL NERVOUS SYSTEM cont.

MAJOR DRUGS (PROPRIETARY NAME IN PARENTHESES)	PURPOSE	ROUTE OF ADMINISTRATION	ADVERSE EFFECTS
Caffeine	Central nervous system stimulant; increases mental alertness, elevates spirits, reduces fatigue	Oral; intramuscular when combined with sodium benzoate	Relatively non-toxic; excessive amounts can cause tachycardia, heart palpitations, irritability, insomnia; may be habituating

* Found on every emergency drug tray.
** Generic name has been changed to phenytoin.

DRUGS THAT ACT ON THE PERIPHERAL NERVOUS SYSTEM

These drugs include neuromuscular blocking agents, which paralyze skeletal muscles by acting at the motor nerve terminals, and local anesthetics, which block conduction of sensory nerve impulses.

MAJOR DRUGS (PROPRIETARY NAME IN PARENTHESES)	PURPOSE	ROUTE OF ADMINISTRATION	ADVERSE EFFECTS
Tubocurarine chloride (also known as d-tubocurarine)	Neuromuscular blocking agent used during anesthesia to achieve muscle relaxation in abdominal and intrathoracic surgery	Parenteral (rapid onset of action)	Hypertension, circulatory collapse, bronchospasm, hypoxia
Succinylcholine chloride (Anectine Chloride)	Neuromuscular relaxant used during anesthesia and electroshock therapy	Intravenous (rapid onset of action)	Respiratory depression; respiratory paralysis
Cocaine hydrochloride (Cocaine)	Local nerve blocking agent; produces surface anesthesia of eye, mucous membranes of nose and throat; no longer administered systemically as highly toxic	Topical	Central nervous system stimulation causing euphoria, excitability, convulsions; followed by depression of central nervous system; may induce psychic dependence as it gives user euphoric "high"
Procaine hydrochloride (Novocaine) ⎫ Lidocaine* (Xylocaine) ⎭	Synthetic local anesthetics used as nerve blocks for regional or spinal anesthesia; lidocaine widely used to treat ventricular arrhythmias	Injection	Dizziness, tremors, convulsions followed by falling blood pressure and respiratory arrest

* Found on every emergency drug tray.

DRUGS THAT ACT ON THE CARDIOVASCULAR SYSTEM

This group includes drugs that act on the blood and the blood-forming organs, drugs that act on the heart, drugs that act on the blood vessels, and drugs used to treat hypertension.

MAJOR DRUGS (PROPRIETARY NAME IN PARENTHESES)	PURPOSE	ROUTE OF ADMINISTRATION	ADVERSE EFFECTS
Ferrous sulfate	Prescribed in iron deficiency anemia	Oral	Gastric irritation, nausea, and diarrhea
Iron dextran injection (Imferon)	Same as above	Deep intramuscular	Itching, headache; in cases of overdosage, hemochromatosis; patients taking iron preparations will have black stools; excessive iron can cause poisoning leading to circulatory collapse

DRUGS THAT ACT ON THE CARDIOVASCULAR SYSTEM cont.

MAJOR DRUGS (PROPRIETARY NAME IN PARENTHESES)	PURPOSE	ROUTE OF ADMINISTRATION	ADVERSE EFFECTS
Cyanocobalamin (also known as vitamin B₁₂)	Contains cobalt; obtained from liver or from cultures of specific microbes; prescribed for pernicious anemia and nutritional anemia	Intramuscular	None have been noted
Vitamin K	Increases coagulation time of blood; administered to stop bleeding; prophylactically, prevents hemorrhage in newborn infants	Intramuscular; oral	Intravascular clotting
Sodium heparin	Used to prolong blood clotting time; prevents formation of new thrombi but does not dissolve existing ones; used when rapid action is desired	Parenteral	Thrombus (or thrombi) can develop if withdrawn rapidly; alopecia and osteoporosis occur rarely with prolonged use; overdose may cause bleeding
Coumarin derivatives	Same as above, except prescribed for long-term anticoagulation	Oral	Excessive bleeding
Digitalis	Commonly prescribed for heart disease; increases strength of cardiac contractions, slows heart rate, depresses electrical activity of heart muscle	Oral usually; may be intramuscular	Dizziness, ringing in ears, nausea, diarrhea; may also cause respiratory depression, cardiac arrhythmias, respiratory arrest
Nitroglycerin	Vasodilator; reduces vascular resistance and lowers blood pressure; counteracts pain due to circulatory disturbance	Sublingually, as it is absorbed quickly through mucous membranes of mouth	Dizziness, weakness, headache
Reserpine	Effective in treating hypertension	Oral usually, but may be administered parenterally	Weight gain, tremors, dizziness, mental depression
Hydralazine hydrochloride (Apresoline)	Same as above	Same as above	Headache, sometimes palpitations, numbness and tingling of extremities, mental depression, anxiety

DRUGS THAT ACT ON THE KIDNEYS

MAJOR DRUGS (PROPRIETARY NAME IN PARENTHESES)	PURPOSE	ROUTE OF ADMINISTRATION	ADVERSE EFFECTS
Furosemide (Lasix)	Diuretic; inhibits reabsorption of sodium, thus greatly increases urinary output; used when more potent diuretic required	Oral	Dehydration, circulatory collapse; patients receiving this drug must be under close medical supervision
Chlorothiazide (Diuril)	Same as furosemide except less potent	Oral	Hypotension, nausea, diarrhea, fatigue, muscle cramps, rash

HORMONES

MAJOR DRUGS (PROPRIETARY NAME IN PARENTHESES)	PURPOSE	ROUTE OF ADMINISTRATION	ADVERSE EFFECTS
Ergot	Increases uterine contractions and constricts uterine blood vessels following delivery of fetus	Oral; parenteral	Tingling, itching, headache, nausea, abdominal cramping, diarrhea, elevated blood pressure
Posterior pituitary (Pituitrin)	Increases uterine contractions, thus used to induce or stimulate labor and control hemorrhage following delivery	Parenteral; buccal where it is absorbed by mucous membranes	Uterine rupture; patients must be under continuous surveillance by medical personnel
Estrogen, progesterone, and synthetic progestins	Used to treat gynecologic disorders; in various combinations, they are effective oral contraceptives	Oral; intramuscular injection	Headaches, nausea, increase in extracellular fluid leading to edema; prolonged estrogen therapy has been linked with increased incidence of cancer of the uterus
Testosterone	Used to treat dysfunction of male reproductive system; in females, prescribed for excessive uterine bleeding, to prevent lactation, in treatment of breast cancer	Oral; intramuscular injection	Decrease in sperm production, increased libido and masculinization in women; gastrointestinal upsets, jaundice
Anti-inflammatory steroids	Administered in rheumatoid arthritis, gout, some skin diseases, allergic manifestations, eye diseases; reason for their anti-inflammatory effect not yet understood	Oral; parenteral; topical; by injection into affected joints and bursae	After prolonged use: fluid retention, facial rounding (moon face), weight gain, menstrual irregularities, elevated blood pressure, skin pigmentation, mental depression or euphoria, delayed wound healing
Hydrocortisone sodium succinate* (Solu-Cortef)	Highly effective in counteracting severe allergic reactions; used for short-term emergency therapy	Parenteral	

* Found on every emergency drug tray.

DRUGS THAT AFFECT METABOLISM

MAJOR DRUGS (PROPRIETARY NAME IN PARENTHESES)	PURPOSE	ROUTE OF ADMINISTRATION	ADVERSE EFFECTS
Insulin	Increases ability to utilize glucose, thereby lowering blood sugar level; aids in conversion of fat to glycogen and promotes protein synthesis; used to control diabetes mellitus; five types, which are prescribed according to onset of action and its duration	Subcutaneous	Rash, tissue atrophy at injection site, coma; patients must be observed closely until their regimen is regulated; any changes in daily living schedules may give rise to severe reaction
Thyroid preparations	Used in treatment of hypothyroidism, cretinism, obesity	Oral	Nervousness, palpitations, tachycardia, sweating, insomnia, tremors, weight loss
Calcium	Used to treat diet deficiency diseases; also to treat tetany	Intravenous; oral	Gastrointestinal irritation; peripheral vasodilatation resulting in fall in blood pressure
Phosphorus	Used to treat diet deficiency diseases	Oral	
Vitamins	Same as for phosphorus	Oral; some B complex vitamins administered intramuscularly	Excessive doses of vitamin A may cause swelling, pruritus, sparse coarse hair

DRUGS THAT ACT ON THE GASTROINTESTINAL TRACT

These include agents that reduce and relieve intestinal spasm, digestants and emetics, and cathartics.

MAJOR DRUGS (PROPRIETARY NAME IN PARENTHESES)	PURPOSE	ROUTE OF ADMINISTRATION	ADVERSE EFFECTS
Sodium bicarbonate* Magnesium hydroxide Aluminum hydroxide	Neutralize gastric acids	Oral, in tablet, powder or liquid suspensions	Overneutralization and rebound secretion, gastric distention
Dilute hydrochloric acid	Prescribed to aid in digestion when supply of hydrochloric acid secreted in stomach is deficient	Oral, either in solution or in capsule form	May damage tooth enamel if not properly administered
Pancreatin	Used as digestive aid; contains some of the enzymes produced by pancreas	Oral	
Apomorphine hydrochloride	Used to induce vomiting in cases of acute poisoning	Subcutaneous injection	
Kaolin Activated charcoal	Absorbents; used in cases of poisoning to delay absorption of poisons until gastric lavage can be performed	Oral	
Cathartics:			
Psyllium hydrophilic muciloid (Metamucil)	Induce evacuation from bowel; bulk cathartic not absorbed but increases bulk in intestinal tract by absorbing gastrointestinal fluid	Oral	*All cathartics:* Dependency; electrolyte imbalance; should not be used in undiagnosed abdominal pain
Magnesium hydroxide mixture	Induces evacuation from bowel	Oral	
Castor oil	Induces evacuation from bowel; irritant cathartic; irritates mucosa of intestinal tract to produce catharsis; frequently prescribed as cathartic of choice before radiologic procedures requiring bowel to be free of fecal material	Oral	
Milk of magnesia	Saline cathartic; prevents absorption of water out of intestinal tract, draws fluid in, thereby increasing bulk	Oral	
Mineral oil	Lubricant cathartic; not absorbed; mechanical aids which lubricate intestinal tract and prevent absorption of water	Oral	
Dioctyl sodium sulfmsuccinate (Colace)	Detergent laxative; acts as "wetting agent" to soften fecal material	Oral	
Bisocodyl (Dulcolax)	Contact laxative; acts directly on the large intestine to increase peristalsis	Rectal suppository	
Diphenoxylate hydrochloride with atropine sulfate (Lomotil)	New synthetic antidiarrheic drugs used to relieve cramping pain of diarrhea and to decrease peristalsis	Oral	Drowsiness, dry mouth, nausea

* Found on emergency drug tray in large ampules for intravenous injection to be used in cardiac emergencies for correction of acidosis

DRUGS THAT ACT ON THE SKIN AND MUCOUS MEMBRANES

These include protectives, soothing substances, antipruritics and astringents. Also included are drugs that act locally on the ear and eye, such as anti-infectives and anti-inflammatory agents in aqueous solution; other local anti-infectives; antiseptics; mercury preparations; antifungal agents; and parasiticides.

MAJOR DRUGS (PROPRIETARY NAME IN PARENTHESES)	PURPOSE	ROUTE OF ADMINISTRATION	ADVERSE EFFECTS
Collodion	Protectives; used to cover skin or mucous membranes to prevent contact with irritating substances	Topical	
Dusting powders			
Demulcents			
Ointments			
Soothing substances	Consist of demulcent materials; also protective and non-irritating; found in forms such as lozenges, stomach mucilages, skin ointments, oils	Oral and topical	
Antipruritics:			
Solutions, lotions, pastes, ointments containing phenol, and tars	Used to combat itching	Topical	
Boric and saline solutions		Topical	
Calamine, cornstarch, and oatmeal baths		Topical	
Hydrocortisone ointments, antihistamines		Topical	
		Oral	In large doses may produce excitement, convulsions, and respiratory failure
Astringents:			
Tannic acid	Used to soothe swollen and inflamed tissues, dry "weeping" wounds, promote healing	Topical	
Witch hazel		Topical	
Benzalkonium chloride (Zephiran)	Antiseptic detergent for use in eye; softens cornea; used to cleanse and apply contact lenses	Topical	
Corticosteroid drugs:			
Bacitracin	Anti-inflammatory drugs for the eye; antibacterial and antifungal agents used in eye	Topical	
Erythromycin		Topical	
Sulfonamides		Topical	
Neomycin	Antibacterial, antifungal, antiseptic for treatment of inner ear infection	Topical	
Polymyxin-B		Topical	
Tyrothricin		Topical	

DRUGS THAT ACT ON THE SKIN AND MUCOUS MEMBRANES cont.

MAJOR DRUGS (PROPRIETARY NAME IN PARENTHESES)	PURPOSE	ROUTE OF ADMINISTRATION	ADVERSE EFFECTS
Sulfonamides	As above (p. 96)	Topical	
Benzethonium chloride		Topical	
Thimerosal (Merthiolate)	Local anti-infectives used for external disinfection of skin and mucous membranes; cleansing surgical instruments and equipment in hospitals and other medical facilities	Topical	
Zinc preparations such as zinc oxide, phenolated calamine lotion		Topical	
Iodine preparations		Topical	
Hydrogen peroxide		Topical	
Hexachlorophene preparations (pHisoHex)		Topical	Should not be used regularly; should not be used on denuded skin; may produce cerebral irritation and convulsions
Triacetin Chloroquinaldol	Antifungal agents	Topical	
Benzyl benzoate	Parasiticides used in treatment of scabies and pediculosis	Topical	
Chlorophenothane		Topical	
Sulfur Ointment		Topical	

DRUGS USED TO TREAT ALLERGIES
These include antihistamines and enzymes.

MAJOR DRUGS (PROPRIETARY NAME IN PARENTHESES)	PURPOSE	ROUTE OF ADMINISTRATION	ADVERSE EFFECTS
Antihistamines:			
Diphenhydramine hydrochloride* (Benadryl)	Blocks action of released histamine; produces sedation of central nervous system; used in treatment of nasal, drug, food, and skin allergies; also to treat motion sickness and radiation sickness due to effects of x-ray exposure	Oral; may be administered parenterally	Drowsiness, dizziness, gastrointestinal disturbances; patients must be warned their reaction time may be affected; driving, flying airplanes, working with machinery may be hazardous after taking these drugs
Enzymes:			
Trypsin crystallized (Tryptar, Parenzyme) Fibrinolysin Streptokinase-streptodornase (Varidase)	Act as catalytic agents in digestion of all foods; used to digest protein in form of dead tissue in wounds and to aid in reabsorption of hematomas	(Trypsin) applied as powder on surface of open wounds; (fibrinolysin) intravenous infusion to treat thrombophlebitis; (streptokinase-streptodornase) may be injected directly into body cavities or applied locally	Hives, itching, pain, increased heart rate if administered parenterally; when administered locally, very few adverse effects have been noted

* Found on every emergency drug tray.

DIAGNOSTIC DRUGS

These include drugs used to aid in medical diagnosis in laboratory and radiologic examinations. In radiology, they are used to improve visualization of the organ being studied by increasing or decreasing the density of the organ to produce the desired contrast. Contrast agents with high atomic weights are called positive contrast agents. Contrast agents with low atomic weights are called negative contrast agents.

MAJOR DRUGS (PROPRIETARY NAME IN PARENTHESES)	PURPOSE	ROUTE OF ADMINISTRATION	ADVERSE EFFECTS
Positive contrast agents:			
Barium Iodine Bromine	Increase organ density; used in barium enema, intravenous pyelograms, gastric and vascular studies; (Iodine) solution of choice determined by need for iodine concentration necessary for study to be done; iodine mixed with sodium meglumine in different proportions; proportions determine viscosity of agent	Oral; intravenous; directly into cavity of body to be studied	Iodine preparations may produce itching, swelling, dyspnea, respiratory arrest; adverse reactions to barium preparations are negligible because they are not absorbed
Negative contrast agents:			
Air oxygen Carbon dioxide Nitrous oxide	Used in pneumoencephalograms, retroperitoneal pneumography, pneumo-arthrography	Pumped directly into area or cavity to be visualized	Oxygen and air may produce gas emboli resulting in chest pain, dyspnea, respiratory failure; adverse reactions to carbon dioxide and nitrous oxide negligible

Methods of Drug Administration

There are three channels by which drugs are administered: topical, systemic, and parenteral. Topical drugs are applied to the skin, and to the eyes, nose, and other orifices of the body. All drugs that are given by mouth (orally), rectum, or inhalation to be absorbed by the body are adminstered systemically. Parenteral drug administration refers to all methods of injection. A drug is administered parenterally when digestive juices would counteract its effect, to produce local anesthesia, and when it is necessary to achieve concentration of the medication at a specific site.

There are five methods of parenteral drug administration, and the RT must familiarize himself with all of them. He must be aware of the sites commonly used and the type and size of needle generally preferred when parenteral medications are ordered.

1. Subcutaneous: injected into the subcutaneous layer of the skin (Fig. 13-1).
2. Intramuscular: injected into the muscular layer through the skin and subcutaneous tissue into the muscular tissue (Fig. 13-2).
3. Intradermal: injected between the layers of the skin (Fig. 13-3).
4. Intravenous: injected into a vein.
5. Intraspinal: injected into a spinal interspace. The site varies according to the puncture to be done.

Procedure for Administration of Medication

ORAL DRUGS

Oral administration of drugs is the safest and most efficient method and is the route most often used. Nevertheless, there are several valid reasons for not giving drugs orally; the drug has an unpleasant taste; the drug causes nausea and vomiting; the drug is destroyed by digestive juices; there is danger of aspiration; the patient is uncooperative; or more rapid absorption is desired. Oral medications are available in liquid, tablet, or capsule form.

When the radiologist desires an oral medication to be given, the RT must wash his hands and assemble a tray, the proper medication, a graduated medicine glass, and a glass of water (if the patient is permitted to swallow water). It is desirable to prepare an identifying ticket which states the patient's name and the drug ordered by the physician, as well as the strength and amount of drug ordered. This ticket is placed on the tray with the medication.

When the RT has prepared the drug for administration, he takes the tray to the radiologist and asks him to read the label on the drug bottle. The RT then pours the desired amount of the drug into the graduated medicine glass. The RT may then be re-

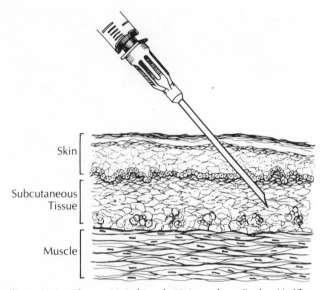

Skin

Subcutaneous
Tissue

Muscle

Figure 13-1.   Figures 13-1 through 13-3 are from Eunice M. King,
Lynn Wieck, and Marilyn Dyer, *Illustrated Manual of Nursing Techniques* (Philadelphia: J. B. Lippincott Company, 1977), pp. 243, 244,
and 242.

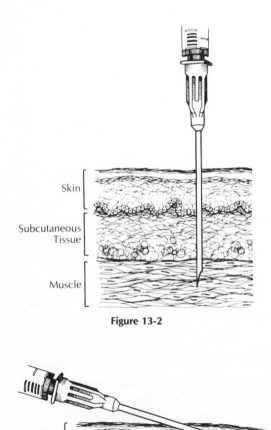

Skin

Subcutaneous
Tissue

Muscle

Figure 13-2

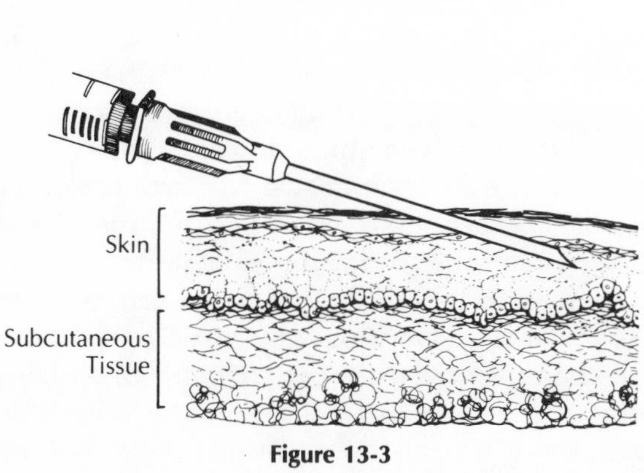

Skin

Subcutaneous
Tissue

Figure 13-3

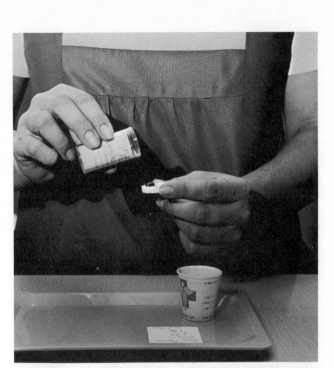

Figure 13-4.   Figures 13-4 through 13-9 are from LuVerne Wolff
Lewis, *Fundamental Skills in Patient Care* (Philadelphia: J. B. Lippincott
Company, 1976), pp. 333, 344-45, 346, 356, and 354.

quested to give the drug to the patient. If so, he once
again identifies the patient and then gives him the
medication (Fig. 13-4). Stay with the patient to be
certain that the drug is swallowed. Offer the patient a
glass of water if it is permitted. Return the tray to the
proper area. Discard the medicine cup or glass and
again wash your hands.

SUBCUTANEOUS MEDICATIONS

These are given at a 45° angle by injection
into the subcutaneous layers. If the radiologist requests that a medication be prepared to be given
subcutaneously, the RT will need a syringe of proper
size (usually 3 or 5 ml.), a needle ⅝ inch long with a
23 to 25 gauge lumen, three alcohol sponges, and the
medication.

Most subcutaneous (sub q.) injections are
given in the outer surface of the upper arm or the
anterior surface of the thigh (Figs. 13-5 and 13-6).

When the correct medication and the equipment are arranged on the tray, the RT may notify the
radiologist. They approach the patient, identify him,
and explain the procedure to him. The RT then may
open the vial and present it to the radiologist with the
label facing him so that he can read it and draw up the
medication. While he is doing this, the RT will expose
an area on the upper arm or the thigh for injection.
The medication is given by the radiologist. The RT
then properly disposes of the equipment and washes
his hands.

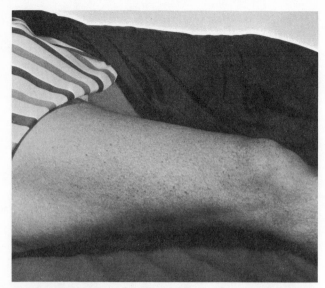

Figure 13-5

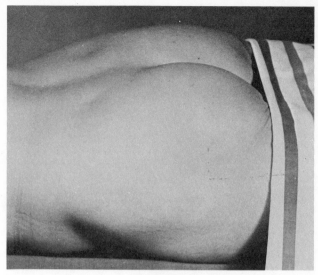

Figure 13-7

dle 1½ inches long is adequate, and the gauge will be 18 to 22, depending upon the viscosity of the medication. A 22 gauge needle should be used whenever possible, because it causes the least pain. The materials required are the same as for the subcutaneous injection, and the procedure is also the same. The usual area for injection of an intramuscular medication is the upper-outer quadrant of the gluteus maximus muscle. (Fig. 13-7). Other areas where an intramuscular injection may be given are the deltoid muscle and the ventrogluteal and vastus lateralis muscle.

While the physician is drawing up the medication, the RT can explain the procedure to the patient and position him for the injection. The patient is instructed to turn to the prone position or to his side (right or left) and the hip is exposed. After the physician has given the injection, return the patient to a comfortable position and dispose of the equipment properly. Wash your hands.

INTRADERMAL INJECTIONS

Intradermal injections are usually given into the inner aspect of the forearm; however, other sites are also acceptable. A very short needle, about ½ inch in length, is used. The lumen of the needle should be approximately 26 gauge. Only very small amounts of medication are given intradermally. They are best measured in a 1 cc. syringe. A tuberculin syringe is desirable because of its very fine calibration. The procedure is the same as for the subcutaneous and intramuscular injection. This type of injection often causes a burning sensation at the site. This possibility should be explained to the patient before the injection is given.

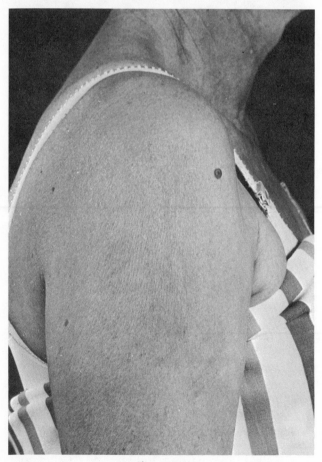

Figure 13-6

INTRAMUSCULAR INJECTIONS

The length of the needle required for intramuscular injections is largely determined by the patient's weight. For the average adult patient, a nee-

INTRAVENOUS INJECTIONS

The routine for intravenous administration of medication varies depending on the type and amount of medication or solution to be administered. Some drugs will be given intravenously (IV) in small amounts, rapidly; others are given over longer periods. If the drug is to be administered rapidly, the RT will select a syringe of the proper size and a needle. The needle is usually 1 inch in length with a lumen varying from 18 to 22 gauge, depending on the viscosity of the solution. If the drug is to be administered over a longer period of time and is in 250 to 1000 cc. of solution, a venous catheter may be preferred. The catheter is made of flexible plastic and is more comfortable and less apt to become dislodged from the vein. Venous catheters are available in various sizes, with an 18 gauge being the usual one for an adult patient. They are mounted on a syringe and threaded with a needle which is removed after the catheter is introduced into the vein. After the syringe and needle are withdrawn from the catheter, the tubing from the intravenous solution is connected to the catheter (Fig. 13-8).

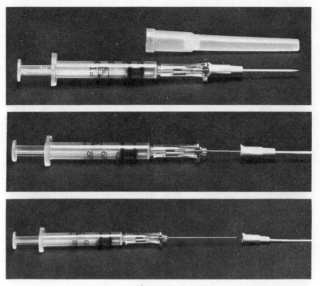

Figure 13-8

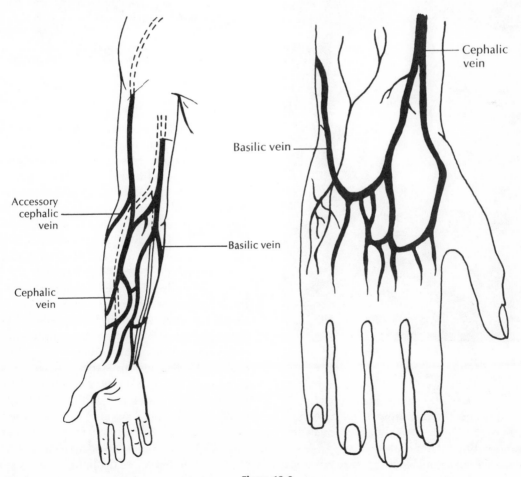

Accessory cephalic vein

Basilic vein

Cephalic vein

Basilic vein

Cephalic vein

Figure 13-9

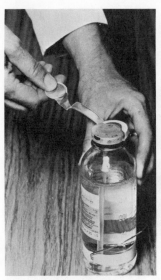
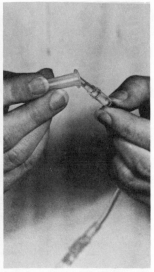

Figure 13-10   Figure 13-11

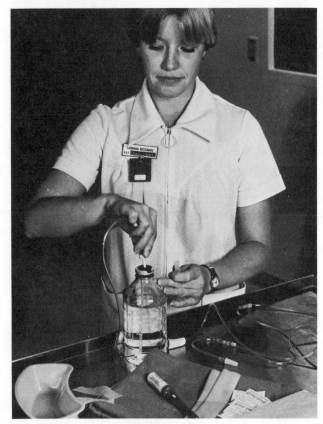

Figure 13-12

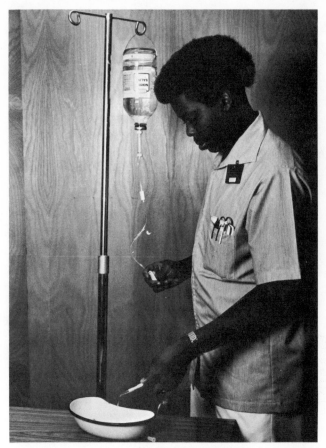

Figure 13-13

flex his arm and will become very uncomfortable. For long-term IVs, veins in the forearm and the back of the hand are recommended (Fig. 13-9).

The type of solution to be administered also influences the vein selection. Hypertonic solutions, those administered rapidly, and thick, sticky solutions should be given into a large vein such as the antecubital vein or another vein of the forearm.

A tourniquet, several alcohol sponges, four strips of adhesive tape, and the proper medication or solution are placed on the tray. An IV standard is placed at the head of the table if it will be needed for holding containers of solutions that infuse slowly. If this is the case, IV tubing will also be needed.

The RT notifies the radiologist when the necessary items are assembled. The procedure is explained to the patient. If the solution to be administered is in an IV infusion container, the RT may remove the metal cap and rubber diaphragm from the bottle (Fig. 13-10). The tubing may be opened and the protective cap may be removed from the drip chamber (Fig. 13-11). The tip of the drip chamber must remain sterile. If it becomes contaminated, replace it. The drip chamber tip is inserted into the rubber stopper (Fig. 13-12). Clamp the tubing with the clamp that

The injection site will vary depending upon the condition of the patient's veins, the medication to be administered, and the duration of the injection. For short-term (not more than one hour) or for a small dosage injection, the antecubital vein, is preferred because it is accessible and easy to enter in most persons. It is not recommended for long-term IV therapy because this inhibits the patient's ability to

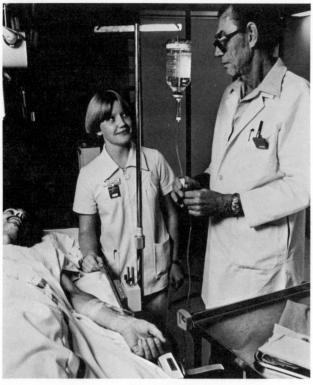

Figure 13-14

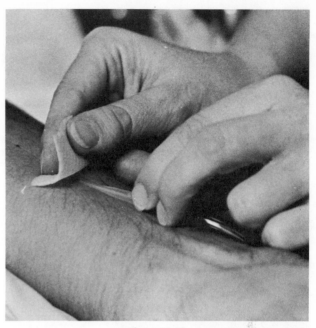

Figure 13-15

comes with it. Have a receptacle at hand. Invert the bottle of solution and hang it on the standard. Remove the protective tip from the end of the tubing. Open the clamp and allow the fluid to run through the tubing until all air is removed (Fig. 13-13). Re-clamp the tubing. Replace the protective tip on the end of the tubing, using aseptic technique. Offer the radiologist the tourniquet and an alcohol sponge. When he has selected the site of injection, hand him a syringe with the venous catheter or proper needle attached. After the medication has been given or the infusion started, make the patient comfortable. Make certain that venous catheters are securely taped in place. The physician will indicate how much time is required for the solution to infuse. This should be noted and the IV monitored so that the timing will be correct (Fig. 13-14).

The rate of infusion (drops per minute) may be controlled by using the clamp to open or close the tubing as desired. The dripmeter at the top of the tubing permits the RT to count the number of drops that enter the vein per minute.

The IV standard should be placed 18 to 24 inches above the level of the vein, because the height at which the container of solution is held affects the rate of flow. If the bottle of solution is placed lower than the vein, blood will flow into the tubing.

If there is a question about the rate of infusion, a safe rule to follow is to allow the solution to

infuse at 15 to 20 drops per minute. If a large amount of solution infuses too quickly, there is danger of fluid intoxication or pulmonary edema. Unless the radiologist has ordered a rapid infusion, the rate of flow of an IV infusing very rapidly should be slowed down.

Any patient complaint of pain or discomfort at the site of injection should be heeded. The site should be checked immediately. Swelling around the site or cold, blanched skin is an indication that the needle or the catheter has become dislodged from the vein and the fluid or medication is infiltrating into surrounding tissues. The RT should clamp the tubing immediately to stop the infusion and notify the radiologist, because tissue damage can be caused by infiltration.

IV medications act very rapidly. Any complaint by a patient of itching or a feeling of congestion or fullness in the chest or throat is cause to discontinue administration of IV medication. *Do not wait* for further evidence of complication. Stop the IV infusion immediately and notify the radiologist.

DISCONTINUING IVs

To discontinue an IV the RT will need alcohol wipes, a scissors, and a pre-packaged narrow bandage such as a Band-Aid. The tape holding the needle or venous catheter in place should be completely removed so that the catheter or needle is free and is visible as it is removed. The clamp should be turned off. An alcohol sponge should be in readiness. Gently withdraw the catheter from the vein until it is entirely removed (Fig. 13-15). Immediately place an alcohol

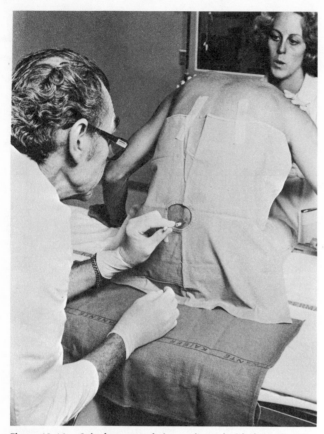

Figure 13-16. Spinal puncture being performed with the patient in a bent sitting position.

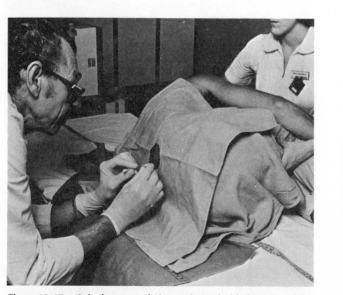

Figure 13-17. Spinal puncture being performed with the patient lying on his side. The RT is assisting the patient to maintain this position. The patient's knees are flexed and his head is brought down close to his knees so that his back will arch.

sponge over the site and apply pressure to that area until the bleeding stops. Then apply the bandage to the area.

If there is a possibility that the venous catheter may have broken off and did not come out of the vein intact, apply a tourniquet above the injection site tightly and notify the radiologist. The IV tubing may be used as a tourniquet.

INTRASPINAL INJECTIONS

These injections are given with a needle 3½ inches long. The lumen is between 20 and 25 gauge. Spinal puncture needles have a stylette that remains in place until the physician has completed the spinal puncture. When the needle is in the desired position in the spinal column, the stylette is removed and the syringe containing the medication is attached to the needle.

Most spinal medications are administered by physicians who are about to perform a special procedure. Myelograms, which are commonly done in the radiology department, involve spinal puncture. There will be a sterile tray opened with the necessary equipment and medications on it. The RT may assist by obtaining extra articles needed by the physician and placing them on the sterile field. The patient is placed in either a bent, sitting position or lying on his side with knees and head as close together as possible so that the back is arched. This makes the spinal column more accessible for puncture (Figs. 13-16 and 13-17).

NEEDLES, SYRINGES, AND MEDICINE GLASSES

Needles range in size from 1½ to 6 inches. The size of the lumen is called the gauge of the needle, and it ranges from sizes 13 to 27. The most common sizes are from 18 to 23, and most needles are from ⅝ to 1½ inches long. Most needles are disposable; however, there are certain special needles made of surgical steel that are cleaned for re-use. The gauge of the needle is printed on the hub of non-disposable needles. Gauge and length of disposable needles are printed on the outside of the wrapper. After use, a disposable needle should be broken or crushed and then discarded. The RT must be careful not to prick himself when handling used needles—a very hazardous hospital accident. Infectious hepatitis may be contracted in this manner.

Most syringes also are disposable. They are available in sizes from 1 to 50 cc. Syringes are calibrated in cubic centimeters and in minims; 1 cc. equals 16 minims. Disposable syringes are prepackaged in paper wrappers, and most often needles are attached. The size of the syringe and the size of the needle are printed on the package (Fig. 13-18). Some

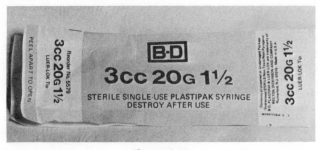

Figure 13-18

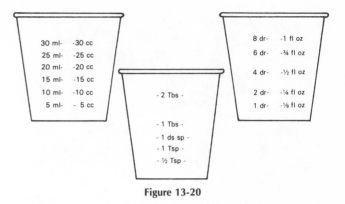

Figure 13-20

syringes are pre-packaged in hard plastic containers, with the size of the syringe and needle printed on the outside of the package. One type of syringe is non-disposable, made of glass; it has a plunger holder and metal control handles. This type of syringe is used for special procedures that require the physician to keep a very firm grip on the syringe. It consists of plunger, barrel, and tip (Fig. 13-19).

After use, a syringe should be rinsed thoroughly and returned to the central supply for recleaning and sterilizing if it is a non-disposable syringe. If it is a disposable syringe, it should be crushed, or the needle should be broken off with the tip of the syringe to prevent re-use.

Most medicine glasses are made of disposable plastic. All are of 1 ounce size and are calibrated for household, apothecary, and metric measures. The RT should know how to convert from one system to another (Fig. 13-20).

INJECTABLE MEDICATIONS

Injectable medications are packaged in ampules, vials, and vacoliters. A vial is a glass container with a rubber stopper circled by a metal band; the band holds the rubber stopper in place. Vials generally are available in 10, 20, 30, and 50 cc. sizes. On the label are found the name of the medication, the dosage per cubic centimeter, and the route by which it may be administered, e.g. morphine sulfate: 1 cc. = 15 mg.

The needle is inserted through the rubber stopper into the solution. The solution runs into the syringe more quickly if air is injected into the vial before the solution is drawn up. The rubber stopper should be wiped with an alcohol pad before the needle is inserted into the vial (Fig. 13-21).

An ampule is always a single dose container and is made entirely of glass. The indented area at the neck is opened by filing the neck with a small metal file (Fig. 13-22). The top then easily snaps off the container. The RT must never attempt to snap the top off an ampule without protecting his hands with a sterile gauze pad, because the glass may break unevenly and cut the hand. The ampule is labeled like

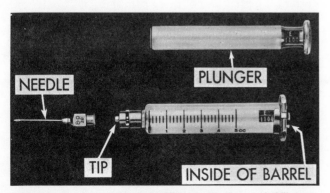

Figure 13-19. From LuVerne Wolff Lewis, *Fundamental Skills in Patient Care* (Philadelphia: J. B. Lippincott Company, 1976), p. 336.

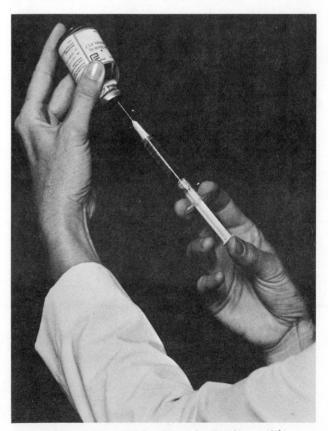

Figure 13-21. Withdrawing medication from a vial.

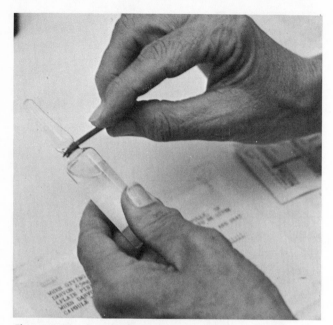

Figure 13-22. From Eunice M. King, Lynn Wieck, and Marilyn Dyer, *Illustrated Manual of Nursing Techniques* (Philadelphia: J. B. Lippincott Company, 1977), p. 233.

the vial, with the name of the medication, the dosage per cubic centimeter and the route of administration printed on the label. If all of the medication is not used, the remainder must be discarded because it does not remain sterile once the ampule has been opened.

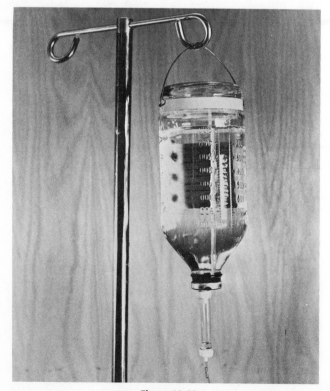

Figure 13-23

The vacoliter is a glass bottle that has been filled under vacuum pressure; it is available in sizes of 250, 500, and 1,000 cc. Like the vial, it has a rubber stopper surrounded by metal. A spot marked "x" inside a circle on the rubber stopper indicates the place where the drip chamber is to be inserted into the bottle. This must be done by firmly pushing into the stopper. After the drip chamber has been inserted, the bottle is inverted for use. The name and quantity of solution is stated on the label. The vacoliter is calibrated in cubic centimeters or milliliters so that the quantity of solution being infused may be easily monitored (Fig. 13-23).

The RT must remember that sterile technique is required for all parenteral medications. If a needle or syringe or the medication itself becomes contaminated, it must be replaced, and the needles must remain covered except for withdrawal of medication until they are used.

Precautions in Drug Administration

All drugs are potentially dangerous. The RT must never become casual or careless when assisting with drug administration and must never give medications on his own authority. The RT must understand the fundamentals of drug administration, in order to assist the radiologist. It is recommended that the RT read all the literature packaged with the drugs used in his department to learn the precautions and contraindications related to the various drugs and the correct method of storing each one.

The patient must be observed during drug administration and for thirty minutes thereafter. Drug reactions occur fairly frequently, most of them during the first thirty minutes if the drug was given orally, intramuscularly, intradermally, or subcutaneously, but are more rapid if the drug was given intravenously. Complaint of itching, shortness of breath, dizziness, or extreme drowsiness should be reported to the physician. The RT must stay with the patient if he has any of these complaints. The patient must not be allowed to drive home by himself after he has received a sedative or a narcotic analgesic, or if he has had a drug reaction.

When preparing medications to be given by the radiologist, read the label carefully. Have the physician read the label before the drug is administered. Check the strength, dosage, and name of the drug. If the RT is requested to record medications given in the radiology department on the patient's chart, he must list the name of the drug, the strength, the amount given, and the route and site. The physician should then sign his name after the recording.

The patient's name should be checked with the medication order to be certain that the right patient is receiving the right medication. Hospital patients will be wearing an identifying name band, which should be read for patient verification. Never use medications from unmarked or poorly marked bottles—these medications should be destroyed. Measure exact amounts of every drug.

If the medication is in liquid form, it should be poured in a direction away from the label on the bottle. If it has formed a precipitate or has changed color, it must not be used. Two medications must not be mixed together unless authorized by the physician. If a mistake is made in drug administration, notify the physician immediately.

Before giving a medication, check the label on the bottle three times—before you measure, before you leave the drug room, and with the physician.

Take only one medication to one patient at a time. Never leave the patient until he has taken the drug offered to him.

FACTORS THAT INFLUENCE DOSAGE

All drugs should be prescribed according to the needs of the individual in question. Every human being is different from every other human being, and each reacts in a unique way to drugs.

Age is a factor in determining the strength and dosage of the drug. The very young and the elderly are particularly sensitive to drugs, requiring far less of any drug than a normal adult dose. In fact, the normal adult dose may be extremely harmful.

Weight and sex are other factors that have a bearing on strength and dose of drugs. In general, smaller doses are prescribed for females than for males.

The individual medication history also influences drug dose. Usually persons who take drugs frequently and in large quantities are less sensitive to drugs than those who rarely or never use them.

Allergy or susceptibility to drugs must be noted and precautions taken. A person's temperament and occupation may also influence his reaction. Questions to be asked are: What is the condition of this patient? Is he young and vigorous? Is he old and weak? Is the patient a child? If so, how old is the child? Why is the medication being given? Does the patient have to be fully sedated, or does he need simply to be relaxed so that the procedure can be properly performed? Obviously, more medication is needed to achieve full sedation than is needed for relaxation.

The time of day influences drug action. A drug given in the morning when a patient is well rested may not be as effective as it might be later in the day. The channel or route of drug administration is also an important factor, as far less medication is required for the intravenous route than for the oral one.

Intravenous drugs are immediately absorbed into the bloodstream and circulated to all parts of the body, whereas oral drugs are absorbed much more slowly, and some of the drug may be inactivated during the period of absorption.

Abbreviations and Equivalents

The following are prescription abbreviations commonly used in hospitals throughout the United States with which the RT should become familiar.

a.c.—before meals
b.i.d.—two times per day
c̄—with
cc.—cubic centimeters
Gm.—gram
gr.—grain
gtt.—drop
h.s.—at bedtime
kg.—kilogram
m.—minim
mcg. or μg.—microgram
mg.—milligram
ml.—milliliter
oz.—ounce
p.c.—after meals
p.r.n.—whenever necessary
q. 4 hrs.—every four hours; q. 2 hrs.—every 2 hours; etc.
q.h.—every hour
q.i.d.—four times per day
ss—one-half
stat.—immediately
suppos.—suppository
tsp.—teaspoon
u.—unit
z—dram
ʒ—ounce

The following measures are used interchangeably in many hospitals. The RT should be able to convert from one to the other immediately.

1 tsp. = 1 fluid dram; z = 4 to 5 cc.
2.2 pounds = 1 kg. (kilogram)
1 inch = 2.5 cm. (centimeters)
30 cc. = 1 oz.
15 cc. = ½ oz.
gr. 1/200 = 0.3 mg.
gr. 1/150 = 0.4 mg.
gr. 1/100 = 0.6 mg.
gr. 1/6 = 10 mg.
gr. 1/4 = 15 mg.
gr. 1/3 = 20 mg.
gr. 1/2 = 32 mg.
gr. 1 = 60 mg.
gr. 15 = 1 Gm. = 1,000 mg.

Summary

The RT is not permitted by law to administer drugs. However, he will be called upon to assist with drug administration. Any person who assists with administration of drugs must know the hazards of drug administration and the precautions that must be taken. He should also have a basic knowledge of drugs and drug action.

Drugs may be classified in several ways. In this chapter, they have been classified according to their actions on the body systems. The drug categories are as follows: antibiotics; drugs that act on the autonomic nervous system; on the central nervous system; on the peripheral nervous system; on the cardiovascular system; on the genitourinary system; on the gastrointestinal system; on the skin and mucous membranes; and on the metabolism. Hormones, diagnostic drugs, and drugs used to treat allergies are included also.

Drugs have generic names, chemical names, and proprietary or trade names. A drug may be marketed under several proprietary names, but its chemical name and its generic name will always be the same.

There are three channels of drug administration: topical, systemic, and parenteral. Topical drugs are applied externally. Systemic drugs are given orally, rectally, or by nebulizer for inhalation. Parenteral drugs are administered intramuscularly, intravenously, subcutaneously, intradermally, and intraspinally.

Drugs administered parenterally induce more rapid reaction than the others, and sterile technique must be followed. Needle size is based on the size of the patient and the specific form of administration. Syringe size depends upon the quantity of drug to be administered.

Medications for parenteral use are packaged in vials, ampules, and vacoliters. The name of the drug, the route of administration, and the quantity per cubic centimeter are listed on the label of the bottle or vial.

All drugs are potentially dangerous and may be life-threatening. The RT must always take every necessary precaution when assisting with drug administration. The right patient must receive the right dose at the right time. The patient must be observed for thirty minutes following administration of a drug. Any symptom of an unfavorable drug reaction must be reported to the physician immediately, and the patient must not be left alone if this has developed. Patients who have received a sedative or had a drug reaction must not be allowed to drive home by themselves.

The patient's age, weight, sex, previous habits, allergy and susceptibility, temperament, occupation, and overall physical condition; the reason for administration of the medication; and the time and route of administration are all factors that must be taken into account in determining the strength and quantity of medication to be given. The RT must be aware of these factors and be alert to any deviation from normal reactions to drugs received by patients when in the radiology department.

See Appendix for pre-post test on Chapter 13.

Isolation Technique

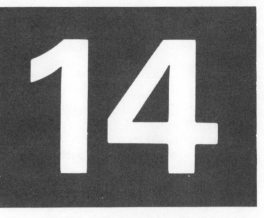

14

Goal of This Chapter

The RT will learn to use isolation technique so that when he is working with patients who have a contagious disease, he may control its spread.

Objectives

When the student has completed this chapter, he will be able to:

1. List the routes of transmission of microorganisms.
2. Define reverse isolation technique and give the reasons for its use.
3. Describe the action an RT would take if he suspects that a patient coming to his department has an infectious disease.
4. Demonstrate, in the laboratory, how to prepare to enter and leave an isolation room.
5. Demonstrate, in the laboratory, how an RT would transport a patient with a contagious disease to and from the radiology department.
6. Demonstrate, in the laboratory, how an RT would take a radiographic exposure in an isolation room.

Isolation technique must be followed by all personnel caring for hospitalized patients with communicable diseases. Its purpose is to control the spread of pathogenic microorganisms from one person to another. When dealing with a patient who has a communicable disease, the RT will be required to use isolation technique both in the patient's room and in the radiology department. He must conscientiously learn and use the proper method, because if the technique is broken, pathogenic organisms can then infect himself, as well as other patients or personnel.

Routes of Transmission of Microorganisms

The spread of microorganisms was discussed briefly in Chapters 2 and 10, and is described more fully in this chapter. Animals, plants, and inanimate objects are reservoirs of infection, as will be described. There are four specific routes by which microorganisms are transmitted.

CONTACT

The contact may be direct, indirect, or by droplet spread. *Direct contact* involves the touching of a person or an animal with an infectious disease. Kissing and sexual intercourse frequently provide the direct contact involved in transmission of pathogens from one person to another. Diseases spread in this manner are infectious mononucleosis, hepatitis A and B, syphilis, gonorrhea, rabies, scarlet fever, and staphylococcal infections.

Glossary

communicable capable of being transmitted from one person to another

contagious capable of being transmitted from one person to another

hepatitis A infectious, short-incubation disease characterized by liver cell degeneration and inflammation

hepatitis B serum, long-incubation disease characterized by liver cell degeneration and inflammation.

infectious caused by or capable of being communicated by infection

isolation unit a cubicle or room set up to sepa-

Glossary cont.

rate persons with communicable disease from contact with other persons

reservoir a person or animal who harbors disease-causing organisms but does not have clinical disease

resistance the natural ability of a normal person to remain unaffected by disease-causing agents in his environment, such as poisons, toxins, or pathogenic microorganisms

---

Indirect contact is defined as the transferring of pathogens to oneself by touching objects that have been contaminated by an infected person. Scarlet fever, measles, mumps, and hepatitis A and B may be spread in this way.

Droplet spread occurs when an infected person coughs or sneezes, spraying the pathogens on a previously uninfected person. Diseases spread in this manner are meningococcal meningitis, measles, chickenpox, pneumonias, influenza, common colds, and mumps.

VEHICLE

A vehicle is a mean of conveyance; thus, with reference to pathogens, the vehicle may be contaminated water, food, medicine, or blood. Typhoid fever, salmonella infections, bacillary dysentery, and hepatitis A may be spread in this way.

AIRBORNE

Certain respiratory diseases are transmitted through the air. Influenza, coccidioidomycosis, and histoplasmosis are diseases spread in this manner.

VECTOR BORNE

An animal or an insect carries the disease organisms, depositing them on or in a person. Malaria, Rocky Mountain spotted fever, and typhus are in this group. Humans and animals may be reservoirs of infection though they do not have the disease. They are known as carriers.

Control of Communicable Disease

There are two methods of controlling contagious disease: by disinfection and by isolation.

To isolate a patient with a communicable disease means to separate him from other people. This may be accomplished by putting him in a private room or in a ward, depending on how the particular pathogenic organisms are spread. If they can be spread only by direct contact, the patient may be isolated within a ward; if by the droplet or the airborne route, the patient must be isolated in a private room. Everything inside an isolation room or unit is contaminated except for designated clean areas.

Disinfection refers to any physical or chemical means of destroying pathogenic organisms. These methods include steam under pressure, boiling, dry heat, open flame, direct sunlight, drying, and very cold temperatures, the most effective being steam under pressure, as explained in Chapter 10. Chemicals in the form of antiseptics and bacteriostatics are also effective to some degree.

If the RT suspects that a patient coming into the radiology department has a communicable disease, the RT must assume responsibility for preventing spread of the pathogenic microorganisms. If the patient is coughing and sneezing, the RT must provide the patient with tissues and a place to dispose of them. He should instruct the patient to cough and sneeze into the tissues and then discard them safely. The patient should be removed from the crowded waiting room to prevent infection of others. The RT who is caring for this patient should put on a gown to protect his uniform and a mask, if he thinks this is necessary. After the patient is cared for and leaves the department, the RT must wash his hands thoroughly and then disinfect the radiographic table, equipment, and anything in the room that the patient may have touched. He should then remove his gown and scrub his hands again.

The RT in the Isolation Unit

It will be necessary for the RT to enter the isolation unit to make radiographic exposures when the patient is unable to come to the radiology department. He must become skilled in maintaining isolation technique for his protection and for the protection of others.

Once inside an isolation unit, the RT must not touch his face or hair. He must handle linens without shaking them. A "clean" area can be created by placing clean paper towels on a table if it is necessary to place "clean" articles in the room. Use clean paper towels or tissue to touch contaminated articles. Handle faucets with a paper towel. If you have an open cut, or have a cold or sore throat, do not care for patients with communicable diseases. Your resistance to infection is lowered and there is a greater chance of contracting whatever disease the patient has.

To maintain strict isolation technique while making a radiographic exposure, the RT will require the assistance of another technologist or member of the ward personnel.

The RT should have his portable machine and the correct number of cassettes prepared before entering the room. A plastic or double thickness cloth case will be needed in which to place each cassette used to protect it from contamination.

The process is as follows:

1. Push the portable radiographic machine into the room. Have a cassette housed in a plastic case and ready for use.
2. There will be disposable masks in a container and gowns just inside the door of the unit near the sink.
3. Remove your watch and any rings you are wearing. Pin them to your uniform or put them into a pocket. If hair touches collar, a cap should be worn.
4. Remove a mask from the container and put it on (Fig. 14-1).
5. Wash your hands.
6. Take a clean gown (gowns should be folded in the same manner as surgical scrub gowns). Hold it at the neck and let it unfold.
7. Put both arms into the sleeves of the gown and work it on. Do not touch the outside of the gown (Fig. 14-2).
8. Use one covered hand to pull on the sleeve and then pull the other sleeve on (Fig. 14-3).
9. Tie the neck ties of the gown. If you touch the outside of the gown or your hair, you must re-scrub (Fig. 14-4).
10. Tie the waist ties of the gown. You are now ready to work (Fig. 14-5).
11. Approach the patient and greet him. Explain what you must do.
12. Place the covered cassette under the patient (Fig. 14-6).
13. Adjust the machine. Make the necessary exposures. You should have as many cassettes prepared as will be needed.
14. When the exposures are made, have your assistant waiting outside the door.
15. Fold the cuff of the protective case back so that the edge of the cassette is free. Do not touch the outside of the pillow case to the cassette.
16. Your assistant should grasp the cassette and remove it from the case (Fig. 14-7).
17. Make the patient comfortable. Untie your waist tie.
18. Scrub your hands (Fig. 14-8).
19. Untie neck ties and mask ties. Hold the mask only by the strings and dispose of it (Fig. 14-9).
20. Remove the first sleeve of the gown by placing your fingers under the cuff of the sleeve and pulling it over the hand (Fig. 14-10).
21. Remove the other sleeve with your hand protected inside the sleeve of the gown (Fig. 14-11).
22. Slip out of the gown and fold it forward so that the inside of the gown is facing outside. If a cap has been worn, remove it and dispose of it (Fig. 14-12).
23. Drop the soiled gown into the receptacle prepared for it (Fig. 14-13).
24. Re-wash your hands and dry them thoroughly. Do not touch faucet handles with bare hands. Use paper towels.
25. Leave the room. Cleanse the portable radiographic machine thoroughly with an antiseptic solution.
26. Wash your hands once again.

Masks are not always worn in isolation rooms. They are worn for reverse isolation, if a disease may be spread by droplet infection or by the air, and when working with a patient who has a draining wound.

Reverse Isolation

Reverse isolation is also called protective isolation. It protects the patient from contamination due to external microorganisms, as in the case of burn patients with denuded skin, patients who have had organ transplants, and infants in critical care nurseries. The technique is similar to aseptic technique as practiced in the operating room. The RT must thoroughly clean his portable radiographic machine before he enters the patient's room. The cassettes should be encased in sterile covers. Sterile gown, gloves, and mask are donned as in sterile technique. The RT must plan his work carefully with an assistant to prevent contaminating the patient. Trips in and out of the reverse isolation room must be kept to a minimum.

Transferring the Patient with a Communicable Disease

Occasionally it is necessary for a patient with a communicable disease to come to the radiology department for radiographs or treatment. Precautions must be taken to prevent infecting anyone else and also to prevent contaminating a room or the equipment.

The patient must be transported by wheelchair or gurney. If he has a respiratory disease, place a mask properly on his face, and wear a gown to protect yourself.

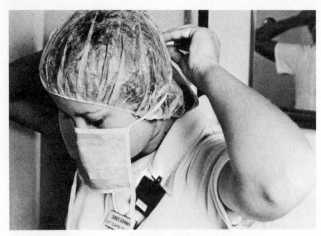

Figure 14-1

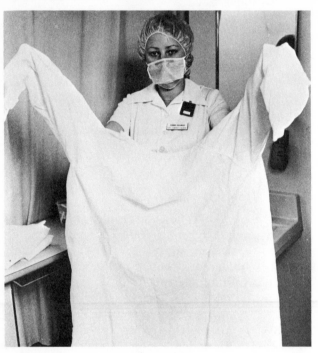

Figure 14-2

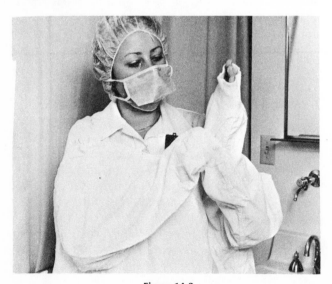

Figure 14-3

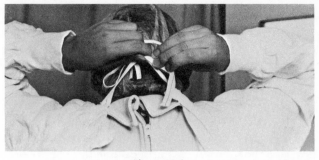

Figure 14-4

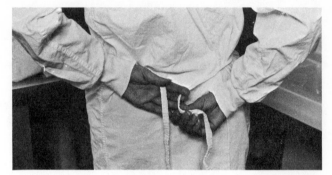

Figure 14-5

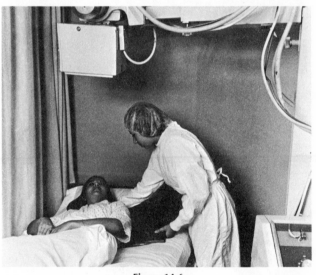

Figure 14-6

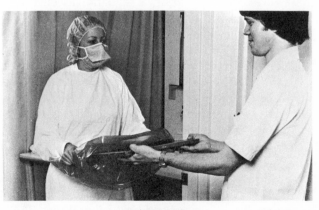

Figure 14-7

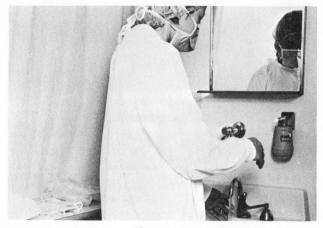

Figure 14-8

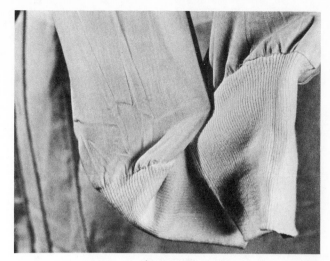

Figure 14-11

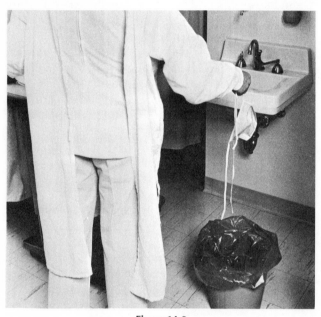

Figure 14-9

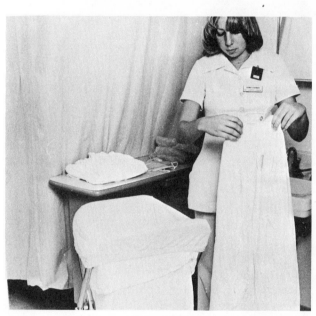

Figure 14-12

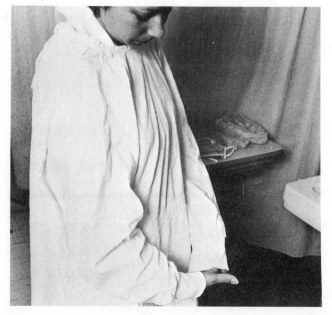

Figure 14-10

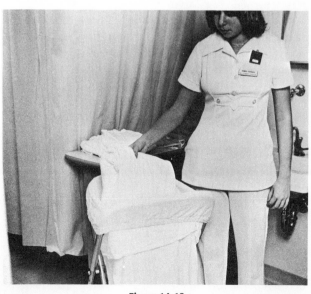

Figure 14-13

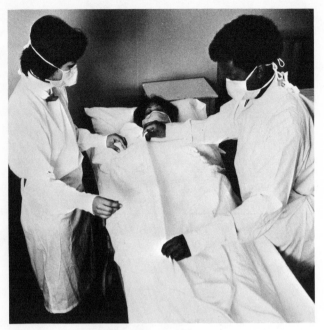

Figure 14-14

Place a sheet on the gurney or wheelchair. Then cover it completely with a cotton blanket. Transfer the patient and wrap the cotton blanket around him (Fig. 14-14).

When the patient arrives at his destination, open the blanket without touching the inside. Place a protective sheet on the radiographic table. Transfer the patient to the table and place a draw sheet over him. Make the necessary exposures. Arrange your work so that the patient does not have to spend any more than the necessary time in the department.

Return the patient to the wheelchair or gurney. Wrap the cotton blanket around him and return him to his room. Notify the ward personnel that he has returned.

In the patient's room, dispose of the soiled sheet and blanket. Wash your hands.

Untie your gown and remove it as instructed in the beginning of this chapter.

Clean the wheelchair or gurney with antiseptic solution. Re-wash your hands.

Return to the radiology department and clean the table and all equipment that was used. Re-wash your hands again.

Summary

Microorganisms are transmitted by contact (direct and indirect), by vehicle, by vectors, or by the air. Methods of controlling communicable disease are isolation and disinfection.

The RT must be prepared to prevent the spread of communicable disease in his own department by isolating a patient who may have an infectious disease, by having the patient cough and sneeze into tissues that are properly discarded, by wearing a protective mask and gown when caring for the patient, and by properly cleaning the room after the patient leaves.

The RT must also learn to maintain strict isolation technique while making radiographic exposures in an isolation unit.

Reverse isolation or protective isolation is necessary when a patient must be protected from pathogenic organisms, because certain patients are particularly susceptible to infections. This technique is used for patients with severe burns, patients who have had organ transplants, and in critical care nurseries. Reverse isolation technique is much the same as aseptic technique used in the operating room.

Transporting patients who have a communicable disease to the radiology department and caring for them there are also the responsibilities of the RT. He must be able to move these patients to and from their rooms and into the radiographic room without infecting other persons or himself.

See Appendix for pre-post test on Chapter 14.

References

Bergersen, Betty S., and Goth, Andres. *Pharmacology in Nursing*, 12th ed. St. Louis: C. V. Mosby, 1973.

Brunner, Lillian Sholtis, and Suddarth, Doris Smith. *The Lippincott Manual of Nursing Practice* 2nd ed. Philadelphia: J. B. Lippincott, 1978.

Cantor, Meyer O. *Instructions for use of Cantor Tube*. Clay Adams, N.J.: Becton Dickinson Co. Rutherford, 1973.

Chabner, Davi-Ellen. *The Language of Medicine*. Philadelphia: W. B. Saunders, 1976.

Committee on Injuries, American Academy of Orthopaedic Surgeons, The. *Emergency Care and Transportation of the Sick and Injured*. Chicago: American Academy of Orthopaedic Surgeons, 1971.

Dorland's Illustrated Medical Dictionary, 25th ed. Philadelphia: W. B. Saunders, 1965.

Frederick, Portia S., and Kinn, Mary E. *The Medical Office Assistant: Administrative and Clinical*, 4th ed. Philadelphia: W. B. Saunders, 1974.

Fuerst, Elinor, V.; Wolff, LuVerne; and Weitzel, Marlene. *Fundamentals of Nursing: The Humanities and the Sciences in Nursing*. Philadelphia: J. B. Lippincott, 1974.

Grant, Harvey, and Murray, Robert. *Emergency Care*. Maryland: Robert J. Brady, 1971.

Hogstel, Mildred. "How to Give a Safe and Successful Cleansing Enema." *American Journal of Nursing*, May 1977, pp. 816-17.

Jacobi, Charles A., and Paris, Don Q. *Radiologic Technology*, 4th ed. St. Louis: C. V. Mosby, 1968.

LeMaitre, George D., and Finnegan, Janet A. *The Patient in Surgery: A Guide for Nurses*. Philadelphia: W. B. Saunders, 1970.

Lewis, LuVerne Wolff. *Fundamental Skills in Patient Care*. Philadelphia: J. B. Lippincott, 1976.

Mager, Robert F. *Preparing Instructional Objectives*. Palo Alto, Calif.: Fearon Publishers, 1962.

McInnes, Mary Elizabeth. *The Vital Signs*. St. Louis: C. V. Mosby, 1970.

Merriam-Webster. *Webster's New Collegiate Dictionary*. Springfield, Mass. G. & C. Merriam Company, 1974.

Musser, Ruth D., and O'Neill, John J. *Pharmacology and Therapeutics*, 4th ed. London: Macmillan Company, 1969.

Picker Radiology Buyers Guide '76. Cleveland: Picker Corporation, 1975, pp. 121, 140, 141.

Sergiovanni, Thomas J., and Carver, Fred D. *The New School Executive: A Theory of Administration*. New York: Mead & Company, 1975.

Snopek, Albert Michael. *Fundamentals of Special Radiographic Procedures*. New York: McGraw-Hill, 1975.

Sutton, Audrey Latshaw. *Bedside Nursing Techniques*, 2nd ed. Philadelphia, W. B. Saunders, 1969.

Thompson, Thomas T. *Primer of Clinical Radiology*. Boston: Little, Brown, 1973.

Vitale, Barbara Ann; Schultz, Nancy V.; and Nugent, Patricia Mary. *A Problem Solving Approach to Nursing Care Plans*. St. Louis: C. V. Mosby, 1974.

Watson, John C. *Patient Care and Special Procedures in Radiologic Technology*, 4th ed. St Louis: C. V. Mosby, 1974.

Wintrobe, Maxwell M., et al. *Harrison's Principles of Internal Medicine*, 7th ed. New York: McGraw-Hill, 1974.

Wood, Lucile A. *Nursing Skills for Allied Health Services*. Vols. 1, 2, 3. Philadelphia: W. B. Saunders, 1975.

Appendix

Pre-Post Test, Chapter 1

1. The following statements describe patients who are entering the radiology department for treatment. Each person feels threatened to some degree because of his impending treatment. Read the statements and determine which need (according to Maslow's hierarchy) might be threatened.
   a. Ms. Alice Bell is a twenty-six-year-old secretary. She has a deforming lump in her left breast. She is to be married in six weeks.
   b. Jamie is a four-year-old. His right arm is injured and he is crying because of the pain of his recent injury.
   c. Mr. Brice is fifty years old. Next year he will be retiring from the job at which he has worked for nineteen years. As he sits in the waiting room, he is occasionally overcome by severe attacks of coughing.
   d. Mr. Bond is forty years old. He has been transported to the radiology department by wheelchair from a hospital ward. He was admitted to the hospital for diagnostic studies of an abdominal mass that was found during a routine insurance physical. He has a small business of his own, a wife, and three young children.
2. A sixty-year-old white female patient enters the radiology department for a barium enema and an intravenous pyelogram. She is extremely pale and thin. Her hands are trembling. When the RT approaches her and asks her to come with him, she gets up slowly, but continues to hold on to her chair. In writing, go through a problem-solving process. Make an assessment of this patient and explain the conclusions that you might reach about how to care for this patient.
3. List four items that an RT should note when he is making a professional assessment of a patient.
4. There is a fellow RT in your department who you are convinced is frequently coming to work drunk. His manner of dealing with patients is often insulting and borders on being abusive. You have reported this to your immediate supervisor, but she has not dealt with the problem. What should you do about this?

Pre-Post Test, Chapter 2

1. Matching: Match the word on the left side of the page with the proper definition on the right.

   h 1. aerobe   a. a cell produced by a microorganism which becomes active under proper conditions.

   c 2. anaerobe   b. a tiny living plant or animal visible only with a microscope.

   g 3. antibiotic   c. does not require oxygen to live.

   f 4. antiseptic   d. a substance that prevents growth of microorganisms.

d 5. bacteriostatic e. disease-producing microorganism.

j 6. medical asepsis f. a substance used to destroy pathogenic microorganisms.

e 7. pathogen g. a chemical substance which has the capacity to inhibit growth or kill microorganisms.

a 8. spore h. requires oxygen to live.

i 9. sterile i. completely free of microorganisms.

b 10. microorganism j. practice that reduces number and spread of microorganisms.

2. List three ways an RT might spread microorganisms in the radiology department.
3. List three methods of controlling the spread of microorganisms. Which of these is the most effective?
4. In the school laboratory, demonstrate the proper method of handwashing for medically aseptic purposes.
5. In the school laboratory, remove linens from a radiographic table that has been used for a patient with an infectious disease and demonstrate the proper method of cleaning the equipment and the table that was used for this patient.

Pre-Post Test, Chapter 3

1. A patient who is totally paralyzed on her right side comes to the radiology department from a hospital ward. She has an IV infusing in her left arm. Her gown has become wet and must be changed. Demonstrate, in the school laboratory, how you will perform this task.
2. A young woman arrives in the radiology department for a barium enema. She is able to care for herself. Please direct her in preparing for this procedure, in writing. She must undress and put on an examining gown.
3. The paralyzed patient in situation one must use the bedpan for urination. Please demonstrate, in the laboratory, assisting her with this procedure.

Pre-Post Test, Chapter 4

1. List four precautions the RT should take to prevent injury to himself when moving a patient.
2. List three safety measures that the RT must take when transferring and returning a patient to the hospital ward.
3. List four symptoms of circulatory impairment that the RT may observe if his patient has a plaster cast of his lower leg.

4. Demonstrate, in the school laboratory, moving an unconscious patient from a gurney to a radiographic table.
5. Demonstrate, in the school laboratory, or explain in writing how the RT would move a patient back to his hospital bed from a gurney if the patient is in a wet, full leg cast.
6. An elderly patient who is paralyzed on her right side has to remain on the radiographic table for over an hour because of a prolonged examination. Demonstrate the precautions that the RT should take with this patient. Include body alignment and skin care.

Pre-Post Test, Chapter 5

1. List normal body temperature of an adult male or female when taken orally.
2. List normal pulse rate of an adult.
3. List four areas of the body where the pulse rate may be measured.
4. List four methods of administering oxygen.
5. The RT must make radiographic exposures of a patient who is too ill to be brought to the radiology department. A portable unit must be taken to the patient's room. When he gets to the room, the RT observes that the patient is receiving continuous oxygen therapy. Describe how this situation should be dealt with by the RT.
6. In the school laboratory, measure and record the temperature, pulse, and respirations of three classmates.

Pre-Post Test, Chapter 6

1. List four symptoms of anaphylactic shock.
2. A patient in the radiology department is receiving a contrast medium intravenously. The patient begins to complain of itching around her eyes and difficulty in breathing. Describe what action the RT should take in this situation.
3. A patient that the RT has been told is a diabetic comes to the radiology department for a barium enema. After about thirty minutes, the patient begins to feel cold and clammy. He responds very slowly when asked questions. Is this of any significance? If so, explain what the RT should do for this patient.
4. A patient on the radiographic table for a radiographic exposure of the clavicle suddenly becomes cyanotic and unresponsive. What action should the RT take? He is alone in the department because it is late at night.
5. A young girl gets off the radiographic table and starts to walk out of the room. She turns very pale

and begins to lose her balance. What action should the RT take?

6. A large young man is lying in a supine position on the radiographic table. He makes a strange noise and begins to thrash about and froth at the mouth. What action should the RT take?

Pre-Post Test, Chapter 7

1. A four-year-old comes to the radiology department for an intravenous pyelogram. You are the RT who will assist with the procedure. How will you begin your work with this patient?
2. A patient has been in an auto accident and must have radiographic exposures of the skull and neck in the emergency room for diagnosis of his injuries. Describe your method of performing this task.
3. Describe the special care that the RT should take if a patient with acute abdominal distress must have a series of abdominal exposures.
4. Demonstrate in the laboratory a sheet restraint that will restrain a two-year-old for an abdominal exposure.
5. Demonstrate manual restraint of a one-year-old's head.
6. Demonstrate a sheet restraint for an infant that leaves both legs exposed.

Pre-Post Test, Chapter 8

1. A patient arrives in your radiology department for a barium enema. He has come from his home many miles away. After the first instillation of barium, the radiologist sees that he is unable to make a diagnosis on this patient because his bowel has not been properly cleansed. The patient must have tap water enemas until clear before the radiologist can proceed. You are the RT that will give these enemas. Please demonstrate in the school laboratory how you should do this. The Chase doll is your patient.
2. Mrs. Jones is a seventy-four-year-old white female. She has come from her room on the third floor for a barium enema. You are the RT that will assist with the procedure. Explain in writing how you will prepare the patient for this procedure.
3. Mr. Brown has a colostomy. The doctor has ordered a barium enema. You are the RT that will assist with the procedure. Mr. Brown is a strong forty-five-year-old man who has had his colostomy for two years. Please explain, in writing, how you will prepare for and assist with the procedure from beginning to end.

Pre-Post Test, Chapter 9

1. List the equipment that must be assembled by the RT if he is to assist with the passage of a Cantor tube.
2. Mrs. Smith has a Levin tube in place and is having continuous suction. The RT must transfer her to the radiology department. He may discontinue the gastric suction long enough to transfer her. Describe how you, as the RT, will arrange this transfer.
3. A Levin tube has been inserted in the radiology department. After the examination, the radiologist requests the RT to remove the tube. Describe how this should be done.

Pre-Post Test, Chapter 10

1. You are the RT who must go to the operating room to make a series of radiographic exposures. It is a small hospital which does not have radiographic equipment in the operating room. Describe, in writing, the preparations that will have to be made before entering the operating room.
2. The radiologist has scheduled an arteriogram for 10 A.M. in room 6. You are the RT in charge of the department. Since this is a sterile procedure, what preparations would you make beforehand to prepare the room for this procedure?
3. During the arteriogram, some solution spills on the sterile field. Describe, in writing, what this does to the sterile field. How might the RT remedy this?
4. In the school laboratory, demonstrate scrubbing, gowning, and gloving for the operating room.
5. Demonstrate, in the school laboratory, opening a large sterile pack to create a sterile field.
6. The radiologist is "scrubbed" and he asks the RT to get him a #16 French catheter. Demonstrate, in the school laboratory, placing this catheter on the sterile field.

Pre-Post Test, Chapter 11

1. Mrs. Brown is in the radiology department for a radiograph of her ankle. She has an open wound on this ankle which is covered by a large dressing. This dressing must be removed for the radiograph and re-applied after the exposures are completed. The radiologist asks the technologist to do this. Explain, in writing, how to remove and re-apply this dressing and why the techniques that you employ are being used.

2. In the school laboratory, demonstrate preparing the skin for an examination that involves a puncture of the lumbar spine.
3. In the school laboratory, demonstrate removal of a dressing from a draining abdominal wound. Use the Chase doll or another student as your patient.
4. In the school laboratory, demonstrate re-application of a sterile dressing.
5. Explain, in writing, how the skin is draped for a sterile procedure.

Pre-Post Test, Chapter 12

1. Mrs. Bill, an eighty-year-old woman, is to go to the radiology department for a gastrointestinal series. She has been incontinent for several weeks and has a Foley catheter in place. You are the RT who will transport her to the department and assist with her examination while she is there. The doctor says that she may not have her catheter clamped. Please explain, in writing, how you will transport her and care for her catheter while she is in your department.
2. In the school laboratory, demonstrate on the female or male mannequin (depending upon the student's sex) a catheterization procedure. You are to insert a Foley catheter.
3. In the school laboratory, demonstrate removal of a Foley catheter.

Pre-Post Test, Chapter 13

1. Mrs. Alvarez has 250 cc. of Conray solution infusing intravenously. She begins to complain of swelling at the site of infusion. Give a written explanation of how you, as the RT receiving the complaint, would deal with this problem.
2. List five factors that might affect the action of a drug.
3. List three precautions an RT must always take when assisting with drug administration.
4. If you are the RT assisting Dr. Blye with administration of an intramuscular drug, what equipment will you need? List needle size, site to prepare for injection, and precautions that you will take in assisting the physician.
5. Matching: Match the symbol on the left with its proper answer in the right column.
   1. c̄   a. dram
   2. Gm.   b. cubic centimeter

3. q.i.d.   c. with
4. ss   d. ounce
5. ml.   e. four times per day
6. cc.   f. milliliter
7. z   g. one-half
8. oz.   h. gram
9. 30 cc.   i. 1 ounce
10. 15 grains   j. 10 milliliter
11. gr. 1/6   k. 1 grain
12. 60 mgs.   l. 1 gram

6. In the school laboratory, demonstrate the following: include preparation of equipment and site for injection.
   a. Preparation for an intravenous infusion of 250 cc. of medication.
   b. Preparation for a subcutaneous injection.
   c. Preparation for an intramuscular injection.
   d. Preparation for an intradermal injection.
7. Match the word in the left column with the definition in the right.
   1. analgesic   a. increases flow of urine.
   2. emetic   b. decreases nervous excitability.
   3. diuretic   c. an agent that induces vomiting.
   4. sedative   d. a drug that relieves pain.
   5. stimulant   e. a drug that increases activity.

Pre-Post Test, Chapter 14

1. Mrs. Grey is in an isolation unit on Ward 4. She has bronchial pneumonia. Her physician has ordered radiographs of her chest. She is too ill to be transferred to the radiology department. You are the RT who is given this assignment. Describe, in writing, how you will make these exposures.
2. List and define four routes of transmission of microorganisms.
3. In the laboratory, demonstrate transferring a patient who has a respiratory communicable disease to and from the radiology department.
4. In the laboratory, demonstrate entering and leaving an isolation room.
5. You are the technologist who is assigned to make radiographic exposures of baby Jones's chest. Baby Jones is a premature infant in the critical care nursery. Describe, in writing, what special precautions should be taken when making these exposures.

Index